Instructor's Guide
for

Contemporary Psychiatric-Mental Health Nursing
The Brain-Behavior Connection
by
Carol A. Glod

Eileen W. Keefe, RNC, MS
Assistant Professor of Clinical Nursing
Louisiana State University
Medical Center
School of Nursing
New Orleans Louisiana

F. A. Davis Company
1915 Arch Street
Philadelphia, PA 19103

Last digit indicates print number: 10 9 8 7 6 5 4 3 2 1

Copyright © 1998 by F. A. Davis Company. All rights reserved. This book is protected by copyright. No part of it may be reproduced, stored in a retrieval system, or transmitted in any form or by any means, electronic, mechanical, photocopying, recording or otherwise, without written permission from the publisher.

Printed in the United States of America

ISBN 0-8036-0294-4

TABLE OF CONTENTS

Contributors

Preface

UNIT 1: INTRODUCTION TO PSYCHIATRIC NURSING

UNIT II: ETIOLOGIC THEORIES OF MENTAL ILLNESS

UNIT III: TREATMENT AND THERAPIES

UNIT IV: PSYCHIATRIC DISORDERS

UNIT V: PROBLEMS IN THE COMMUNITY

UNIT VI: FUTURE CHALLENGES TO DELIVERING CARE TO THE MENTALLY ILL

❏ ❏ ❏ ❏ ❏ **CONTRIBUTORS**

Catherine Caston, PhD, RN
Loyola University-New Orleans
City College-Nursing Program
Assistant Professor
Family Nurse Psychotherapist

Sue C. DeLaune, MN, RN.,C
President, S. DeLaune Consulting
Mandeville, Louisiana.

Angela Frederick, MN, RN.,CS
Assistant Professor of Clinical Nursing
Louisiana State University Medical Center
School of Nursing
New Orleans, Louisiana

Mary Little-Green, MN, RN.,C
Nursing Supervisor
Booker T. Washington
School-Based Health Clinic
New Orleans, Louisiana

Carolyn Mosley, PhD, RN
Associate Professor of Nursing
Louisiana State University Medical Center
School of Nursing
New Orleans, Louisiana

Connie M. Morgan, MS, RN.,C
Assistant Professor of Clinical Nursing
Louisiana State University Medical Center
School of Nursing
New Orleans, Louisiana

Nancy Rankin, MS, RN
Associate Professor of Nursing
Louisiana State University Medical Center
School of Nursing
New Orleans, Louisiana

Georgia Johnson, MS, RN., CNAA, CPHQ
Clinical Nurse Specialist/Director of Quality Support Services
Southeast Louisiana Hospital
Mandeville, Louisiana

PREFACE

This Instructor's Guide is intended to be used with ***Contemporary Psychiatric- Mental Health Nursing: Tthe Brain-Behavior Connection***, by Carol A. Glod. It includes case presentations that are followed by a set of critical thinking issues designed to raise the student's curiosity and level of awareness . Proposed and recommended student activities within the guide include class discussion, small group activities, literature searches, word-find puzzles, cross-word puzzles, and Internet searches. Transparency masters are also provided.

CHAPTER 1: Contemporary Psychiatric-Mental Health Nursing

Case Presentation

Ms. A., a 25-year-old single client, has received psychiatric care for the past 18 months since her elderly parents were killed in an automobile accident. She claimed that she had been hospitalized twice during that period of time because of feelings of guilt, irritability, anger and because she had no one to share in the grieving process. She had no close friends, and her only sibling lived 2000 miles away. She stated that if she had been available to support her parents, they might still be alive. Three months ago, she sought psychiatric care from a clinical nurse specialist (CNS). She stated that she received treatment for sleep disturbance, emptiness, and fear that her sibling would be the next person to die. She characterized her outpatient sessions as brief psychotherapy to help her resolve the multiple problems and feelings of depression surrounding her parents' deaths. She reported that her symptoms diminished at the completion of the psychotherapy sessions, during which the CNS emphasized her strengths and helped her to achieve a higher level of wellness. Within 5 months Ms. A. returned to the CNS, complaining of anxiety, inability to function, and increasing isolation from the workplace. After a complete physical and psychological assessment, no biological conditions were found that could be attributed to Ms. A.'s psychiatric illness. The CNS prescribed lorazepam (Ativan), 1 mg every 4 hours as needed, for the relief of anxiety. The CNS determined that Ms. A.'s inability to complete the grieving process was due to the absence of a social support system. The nurse is aware that some forms of mental illness are situational and that a change in the social aspects of the environment may improve Ms. A.'s outlook. The CNS used a gentle and supportive approach to help Ms. A. reconstruct the memories and to elicit both positive and negative feelings toward her parents and their deaths.

Critical Thinking Issues

1. Examine attitudes and bias toward mental illness.

2. Discuss the role of the nurse psychopharmacologist.

3. Determine the nurse psychopharmacologist's legal responsibility to the client under his or her care.

4. Discuss the role of the CNS in health promotion.

5. What levels of prevention are evident in the case presentation?

6. What factors account for the client's reaction to grief?

7. Discuss how social factors may affect mental health or mental illness.

8. When using the classification system based on DSM-IV, what would be an appropriate Axis I diagnosis for the client in the case presentation?

9. What would be the most appropriate nursing diagnoses for the client?

Student Activities

Word-Find Puzzle

Hidden below are words related to Chapter 1. Circle each word that you find. The words may be found by searching across, up, down, forward, and backward.

ADVOCACY	ETHICAL	MEDICATION	RESTRAINTS
INTERPERSONAL	DSM-IV	MILIEU	ROY
CASE manager	LEGAL	NURSE	SECLUSION
MANAGED care	COMMUNITY	OREM	SECONDARY
MARTHA ROGERS	ECT	PEPLAU	PRIMARY
COLLABORATION		Tertiary	

```
A T I O S C A S E W U A L P E P L L R E N A L A
T A L S E E S R U N P D S M I V H A L W P E P S
M L A C I H T E G J W A Q E R Y O R S L P U N R
I O P U A Y T G W Z H P A N L C O I P T R I R M
L A G E L A V O B N L T A Y R A M I R P E S I A
I N T E R P E R S O N A L E Y C A L K J A E T N
E N T E R O W A I O T T C E U O L L E H O A L A
U N I R E W A H S S P I O H G V A W E N R P N G
Y R A I T R E T W Q U O K V C D A M P R E M E E
S E C O N D A R Y L L N O I T A C I D E M A R D
A U N C O L L A B O R A T I O N O I S U L C E S
T R Y T I N U M M O C B C F H L M P A E L W O A
```

3

PUZZLE SOLUTION

```
A T I O S C A S E W U A L P E P L L R E N A L A
T A L S E E S R U N P D S M I V H A L W P E P S
M L A C I H T E G J W A Q E R Y O R S L P U N R
I O P U A Y T G W Z H P A N L C O I P T R I R M
L A G E L A V O B N L T A Y R A M I R P E S I A
I N T E R P E R S O N A L E Y C A L K J A E T N
E N T E R O W A I O T T C E U O L L E H O A L A
U N I R E W A H S S P I O H G V A W E N R P N G
Y R A I T R E T W Q U O K V C D A M P R E M E E
S E C O N D A R Y L L N O I T A C I D E M A R D
A U N C O L L A B O R A T I O N O I S U L C E S
T R Y T I N U M M O C B C F H L M P A E L W O A
```

1. Divide students into two approximately equal groups, with one group representing the role of the generalist, and the other, the role of the specialist. Within these major groups, subdivide the students into groups of three or four. Assign each subgroup a task of listing and analyzing the responsibilities of the major roles they represent. Ask each student subgroup, through a previously selected recorder, to share its findings with the larger group.

2. Generate a class discussion about the legal and ethical issues related to admissions to and discharges from a psychiatric inpatient facility.

Conceptual Models—Value to Psychiatric– Mental Health Nursing

- Callista Roy—Adaptation

- Martha Rogers—Science of Unitary Human Beings

- Dorothea Orem—Self-care

- Hildegard Peplau—Interpersonal Relationships

Definitions

- Mental Illness—disturbance in an individual's thinking, emotions, behaviors, and physiology

- Mental Health—a state of well-being in which individuals function well in society and are generally satisfied with their lives (ANA, 1994)

Roles of the Psychiatric Mental Health Nurse in Contemporary Mental Health Care

- Generalist

- Specialist

- Primary Care Nurse

- Collaborative Member of the Interdisciplinary Team

- Mental Health Promotion

- Case Manager

- Therapeutic Milieu Director or Manager

- Psychiatric Consultant–Liaison Nurse

- Psychotherapist

- Psychopharmacologist

<u>Legal and Ethical Issues</u>

- Confidentiality

- Admission to a Psychiatric Inpatient Facility

- Discharge from a Psychiatric Inpatient Facility

- Duty to Warn

- Individual Rights

- Informed Consent

- The Right to Refuse Treatment from a Nurse

- Seclusion and Restraints

- Client Advocate

CHAPTER 2: The Nursing Process in Psychiatric–Mental Health Nursing

Case Presentation

A 26-year-old female professional secretary, who was recently unemployed, sought help at the community mental health center. She has a history of psychiatric symptoms, including psychotic and depressive features. She has had two previous hospitalizations, and since the last hospitalization 2 years ago, she has developed obsessive-compulsive features. She has described herself as being a perfectionist and fearful of making mistakes. Upon encouragement from her family, she presented herself for reevaluation and possibly for a change in her treatment regimen. She described her mood as unpleasant and was extremely anxious with "butterflies in her stomach." She had some feelings of inadequacy; a decline in self-worth; and obsessional ruminations that involved dissatisfaction with her marriage, social withdrawal, and inability to experience life's pleasures. She also lacked energy and had a diminished appetite.

She began to sob when reflecting on her life's interruptions and her refusal of invitations to professional and social events. She stated that her work productivity was declining; she found it difficult to make decisions; and she was unable to finish her work assignments. She indicated that termination was the result of these deficits, and she was feeling frustrated, hopeless, and occasionally suicidal. Her affect was flat, and she expressed herself at a normal rate and tone. She was alert and oriented. She denied hallucinations in all five senses. When questioned further about her suicidal thoughts and if she had a plan, she stated, "I plan on using my friend's gun because that will take care of me in a hurry." The client agreed to a voluntary admission to a psychiatric hospital for her protection. After the client was admitted to the hospital, the staff took precautions to make the unit safe. She refused to accept all psychotropic medications that were prescribed because they caused akathisia. She perceived the nursing team to be incompetent. Her level of functioning remained impaired until a clinical nurse specialist was consulted. Through nurse-client interaction, rapport was gradually established and the client's progress slowly improved. A trial of medications was introduced, and eventually an acceptable one was found.

Critical Thinking Issues

1. Identify the problem areas for this client.

2. How important is it to identify the strengths of the client? How can strengths be used as part of the therapeutic process?

3. What are the possible risk factors associated with the care of this client?

4. From the data presented, what nursing diagnoses are most accurate for this case situation?

5. Identify two nursing strategies for each diagnosis.

6. Identify possible outcomes derived from the diagnoses.

Student Activities

Classroom Activity

1. Ask each student to choose a partner and perform and document a mental status examination using the Instructions for Administration of Mini–Mental Status Examination from the <u>Contemporary Psychiatric–Mental Health Nursing</u> text located in Chapter 2.

2. Using the preceding case study and the components of the nursing process, complete a comprehensive nursing assessment.

3. From the data collected, develop three nursing diagnoses using the North American Nursing Diagnosis Association (NANDA) list of approved nursing diagnoses.

a._____

b._____

c._____

4. Develop goal-oriented interventions.

a._____

b._____

c._____

d._____

5. Provide expected outcomes that are derived from the short- and long-term goals.

a._____

b._____

c._____

d._____

6. Formulate an objective outcome that could be tracked to indicate improvement in the client's mental health.

a. _____

b. _____

c. _____

d. _____

Nursing Process

- Assessment

- Nursing Diagnosis

- Outcome Identification

- Planning

- Implementation

- Evaluation

Components of the Mental Status Examination

- General Appearance, Behavior, and Attitude

- Attention and Concentration

- Orientation

- Memory

- Language Function and Characteristics of Speech

- General Intellectual Functioning and Memory

- Cortical and Cognitive

- Functions—Mood and Affect

- Thought Content—Preoccupations and Experiences

- Insight

- Judgment

CHAPTER 3: Therapeutic Relationship and Effective Communication

Case Presentation

A graduate level nursing student assigned to a community mental health clinic for 6 weeks chose to work with a 32-year-old female client who was sexually abused as a child. The student and client contracted for 1 hour twice a week for the duration of the assigned time. During the first session, the client was in a state of anxiety and emotional upset because her relationship with her boyfriend was deteriorating. She described her interpersonal situation as stormy and abusive physically, sexually, and emotionally. The client described her abuse in great detail and cried during each session that the graduate student and she spent together. Occasionally, the client asked the student about her interests, goals, and achievements. Little was accomplished therapeutically during the time they interacted, and because of this the client decided to terminate the contract. Upon learning about the client's decision, the student was surprised and upset to find that she would not be returning to the clinic. The student telephoned the client's home to offer her services. The client was hesitant but accepted, and the student went to the person's home several days later. The client felt that someone finally cared about her and was more willing to share the many painful experiences and feelings brought about by the abuse. The student was reliving her own experiences that she suffered at the hands of her stepfather. She remembered her feelings of abandonment, anger, and fear when her mother refused to acknowledge that her daughter was being sexually abused. She felt that her mother was not willing to protect her from the abusive stepfather. Reliving these memories made it almost impossible for the student to help the client because she was so involved in her own feelings that she was unaware of her client's real concerns. The sessions were terminated, and the client was referred to a clinical nurse specialist.

Critical Thinking Issues

1. Discuss the barriers to communication.

2. Discuss the pros and cons of a communication contract.

3. Discuss the difference between a therapeutic and nontherapeutic relationship.

4. What are the guidelines for establishing boundaries?

5. What phases of the nurse-client relationship were accomplished?

6. What level of communication was established?

Student Activities

Phases of the Therapeutic Relationship

There are four stages of relationship development.

a. Preinteraction Phase
b. Orientation Phase
c. Working Phase
d. Termination Phase

Match the phase of therapeutic relationship between the client (Mr. B.) and the student nurse (Miss S.).

_____ 1. "Mr. B., I don't think I understand what you are saying."

_____ 2. "Mr. B., I'm Miss S., a student nurse and I'll be working at the clinic today."

_____ 3. Miss S. examines her feelings about working with psychiatric clients.

_____ 4. "Mr. B., it is time to review your progress and your unresolved problems."

_____ 5. "Mr. B., tell me more about what you are thinking."

_____ 6. "Mr. B., I'll respect you if you are unable to share your feelings today."

_____ 7. " Mr. B., tell me about your strengths."

_____ 8. "Mr. B., you are welcome to return for help if it is ever necessary."

_____ 9. "Mr. B., you look angry. Tell me about your problem."

_____ 10. "Mr. B., it is important to set goals."

_____ 11. "Mr. B., have your goals been met to your satisfaction?"

_____ 12. "Mr. B., what are your thoughts about changing your behavior?"

Answers to the Phases of the Therapeutic Relationship

There are four stages of relationship development.

a. Preinteraction Phase
b. Orientation Phase
c. Working Phase
d. Termination Phase

Match the phase of therapeutic relationship between a client Mr. B. and the student nurse Miss S.

c_____ 1. Mr. B., "I don't think I understand what you are saying."

b_____ 2. Mr. B., "I'm Miss S. a student nurse and I'll be working at the clinic today."

a_____ 3. Miss S. examines her feelings about working with psychiatric clients.

d_____ 4. "Mr. B., it is time to review your progress and your unresolved problems."

c_____ 5. "Mr. B., tell me more about what you are thinking."

b_____ 6. "Mr. B., I'll respect you if you are unable to share your feelings today."

b_____ 7. " Mr. B., tell me about your strengths."

d_____ 8. "Mr. B., you are welcome to return for help if ever necessary."

c_____ 9. "Mr. B., you look angry. Tell me about your problem."

b_____ 10. "Mr. B., it is important to set goals."

d_____ 11. "Mr. B., have your goals been met to your satisfaction?"

c_____ 12. "Mr. B., what are your thoughts about changing your behavior?"

Cross-Word Puzzle:

Therapeutic Nurse-Client Communication

Across

  1. A favorable reception of another person.
  2. Territory surrounding the person that acts as an invisible barrier beyond which others are expected not to trespass.
  8. Hearing with comprehension.
  10. Ensuring safety to clients as they work through trouble spots with new behavior.
  12. Lead phrases or beginning statements that allow the client to set the direction of the conversation (two words).
  14. Kind of posture the interviewer assumes to communicate receptiveness nonverbally and to show that attention is being given to what is being said.
  15. A feeling that conveys genuine curiosity and a desire to know another person.
  16. Act of providing the person with specific facts that will answer questions or dispel misconceptions and help the person to better evaluate the situation (two words).
  19. Contact made by looking directly at the other person.
  20. A technique that allows the person to collect his or her thoughts and reflect upon the topic being discussed. After waiting a reasonable time, the interviewer can prompt the person to reopen the conversation.
  21. Basic posture of involvement in which the interviewer looks squarely at the person being interviewed.
  24. Confirming whether the information is accurate.
  25. Skill in dealing with persons in a delicate and sensitive manner.
  27. Quality that makes something seem funny or amusing.
  28. Intonation, pitch, or modulation of the voice that expresses a particular meaning or feeling of the speaker.
  29. Act of helping another person.
  30. To show consideration and courteous regard for another person.
  31. Quality of being without bias or prejudice.

Down

1. To believe in and receive favorably.
3. Consent or authorization to behave in new ways.
4. Condition of holding the interview in an area away from the mainstream of activity.
5. Quality of being truthful, upright, or trustworthy.
6. Technique of making attempts to clearly understand a vague, confusing, or unclear message by using a phrase such as, "I'm not sure I'm following what you mean."
7. Letting the person know that his or her feelings are recognized, understood, and accepted while encouraging continued expression of them (two words).
9. Comments are made with interest and concern about observed physical or apparent emotional state (two words).
11. Knowing what to give and when to withhold information.
13. Ethical obligation of nurses to protect matters concerning clients.
17. Kind of questions that do not influence the direction of the client's responses.
18. Nonverbal form of communication through the placement of a hand on another person.
22. Technique that leaves the direction of the conversation to the client. It conveys that the nurse is interested in what will be said next, following verbal responses such as, "Yes," Oh?," or nonverbally by nodding or making facial expressions (two words).
23. Repeating the client's basic statement to the client, providing an opportunity to hear and think about what the client had said.
26. Ability to comprehend how another person feels in his situation and to communicate that acceptance and understanding to him.

DEMENTIA vs. DEPRESSION GRID

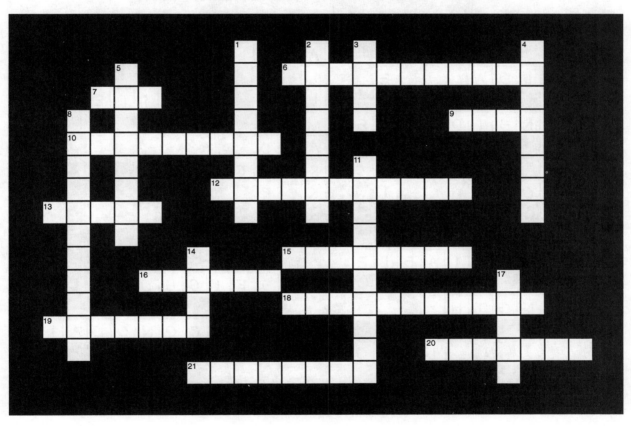

DEMENTIA vs. DEPRESSION

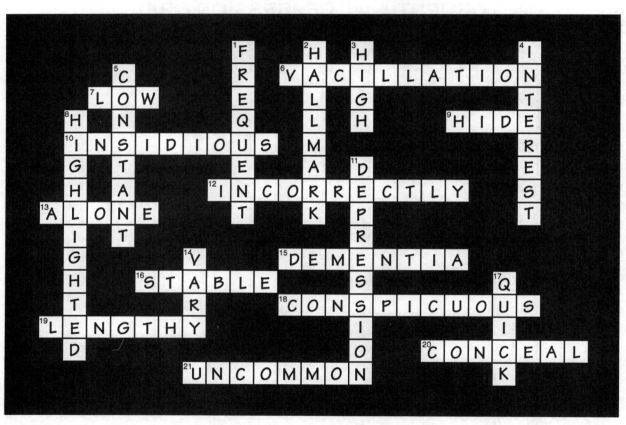

Transparency

Phases of the Therapeutic Relationship

- Preinteraction Phase

- Orientation Phase

- Working Phase

- Termination Phase

Levels of Communication

- Intrapersonal

- Interpersonal

- Small Group Communication

- Organization Communication

Elements of Communication

- The Sender

- The Message

- Verbal Messages

- Nonverbal Messages

- The Channel

  ▾ Visual channel

  ▾ Auditory channel

  ▾ Kinesthetic channel

- The Receiver

- Feedback

- Time and Space

CHAPTER 4: Developmental and Psychological Theories of Mental Illness

Case Presentation

A 10-year-old boy was referred to the community mental health clinic by the school principal for fighting with peers and arguing with his teacher. The school report indicates that the client was enrolled in a regular third-grade class. His grades dropped considerably within the last 3 months, and recent tests reveal that he has a learning deficit. He was recently reassigned to a class that specializes in learning disabilities. The parents told the mental health nurse that they have noticed signs of increased motor activity and learning problems. The boy is easily angered, frequently argues with the parents, blames others for his mistakes, and is unable to accept limits set by the parents. The mother was also concerned that her son disliked the current classroom arrangement, because he threatened to run away from home if things didn't change. The mother reported that her son spends more time alone, and his social skills are inadequate. He refuses to do his homework or household chores, and he does not interact with other family members. When he does interact with his siblings, he becomes verbally abusive and physically violent. He has a limited number of friends, and those who were close to him have been staying away. The mother continued to report that when she attempts to question her son about his friends he becomes extremely agitated and states that his peers are leaving him alone because they don't like him anymore.

Mental Status

The client appeared as a well-nourished 10-year-old who was clean and neatly groomed. He was cooperative, alert, and attentive during the interview. He was oriented to person and place. His general fund of knowledge was less than average, and his vocabulary was limited. His speech was clear, and his judgment was poor. His thought processes were concrete, and attempts to ask questions about his friends and extracurricular activities were firmly resisted by the client. His perception of self-concept was negative. He portrayed a tough-guy image and presented as an individual who was able to take care of himself. The client presented with less than average intelligence and poor school achievement skills, marked emotional regression, and serious maladaptive behaviors that posed a difficulty for his parents.

   His history included aggression toward others, frequent violent outbursts, difficulty in getting along with peers, and noncompliance with adult demands. He experienced internal distress and a sense of deprivation. Developmentally, the client was not yet capable of abstract reasoning. The learning deficits and the increased motor activity are possibly suggestive of some mild underlying neurologic disorder. This may have served to exacerbate symptoms by contributing to his frustration with school and to his poor task mastery.

Critical Thinking Issues

1. Using Freud's psychoanalytic theory, discuss the stage of development exhibited by the 10-

year-old client.

2. Examine the aforementioned scenario using Erikson's theory of personality development.

3. Assess the cognitive development of the 10-year-old client using Piaget's theory.

4. Examine the interpersonal level of development relative to Sullivan's framework.

5. Discuss the problematic behavior of the 10-year-old using one of the behavioral theorist concepts.

6. Discuss the developmental shifts and turmoil exhibited by the 10-year-old client.

7. What is the influence of developmental and psychological theories on the nurse-client relationship in this case?

Student Activities

Directions: Freud's psychosexual theory has six stages. Match the task and the key concepts with each stage. An example has been provided to help you get started.

Psychosexual Stage	Tasks	Key Concepts
Oral	Satisfaction and anxiety management through oral gratification activity	Pleasure is obtained through oral activity.
Anal		
Phallic		
Oedipus complex		
Latency		
Genital		

Answers to Freud's Psychosexual Theory

Psychosexual Stage	Tasks	Key Concepts
Oral (birth to 12 months or longer)	Satisfaction and anxiety management through oral gratification activity.	Pleasure is obtained through oral activity.
Anal (1–3 years)	The child takes particular interest and concern with the process of evacuating bowels and the sensations connected with the anus.	The libidinal energy shifts from the oral cavity to the anus. The pleasurable part of the task is called *anal eroticism.*
Phallic (2½–6 years)	The sexual interest, curiosity, and pleasurable experience center on the genitalia.	The focus has shifted from the excretory organs to the child's own body.
Oedipus complex (4–6 years)	Represents a time of inevitable conflict between the child and the parents. The boy develops resentment and fear toward the father.	If the child desexualizes the relationship with both parents and the process is successful, the child's personality is more definitely shaped.
Latency (6–12 years)	The libidinal energy is not focused on any one area. The child develops skills to help with the transition from the home to a broader environment.	The characteristics of the child are stable behavior and even temperament.
Genital (12–18 years)	A reawakening of sexual interest occurs, and a satisfactory heterosexual relationship is achieved.	Pleasure is obtained through sexual relationships.

Student Activities

Directions: Erikson's Life Cycle Theory has eight stages. Identify the stages and describe the tasks and concepts that occur during the psychosocial stages.

Age	Psychosocial Stages	Tasks	Concepts
0–2 years	Infancy	Trust vs. Mistrust	Develop a sense of trust and view others as trustworthy
2–4 years			
4–6 years			
6–12 years			
13–18 years			
19–-45 years			
46–65 years			
65 years and older			

Answers to Erikson's Life Cycle Theory

Age	Psychosocial Stages	Tasks	Concepts
0–2 years	Infancy	Trust versus Mistrust	Develops a sense of trust and views others as trustworthy.
2–4 years	Toddler	Autonomy versus Shame and Doubt	Develops independence and a favorable concept of oneself.
4–6 years	Early Childhood	Initiative versus Guilt	Realization of a sense of purpose in life and a sense of comfort with one's gender.
6–12 years	School Age	Industry versus Inferiority	Develops a sense of competence.
13–18 years	Adolescence	Identity versus Identity Diffusion	Emancipates self from parents and searches for a sense of identity. Broadens the social sphere.
19–45 years	Young Adult	Intimacy versus Isolation	Shares self with others or, because of fear, develops a sense of isolation.
45–65 years	Middle Years	Generativity versus Self-absorption	Adult is productive, creative, and involved in community activities. Transmits values to the next generation.
65 years and older	Maturity	Integrity versus Despair	Accumulation of wisdom. Experiences love and respect for mankind. Recalls past experiences.

Student Activities

Directions: Erikson's eight stages of development have positive and negative outcomes. Match the following verbal statements with the appropriate outcome.

a. Mistrust	e. Inferiority	i. Shame	m. Identity	
b. Autonomy	f. Integrity.	j. Isolation	n. Guilt	
c. Intimacy	g. Self-absorption	k. Initiative	o. Industry	
d. Despair	h. Identity diffusion	l. Generativity	p. Trust	

Verbal Statements	Outcomes
1. "I will gladly be the spokesperson for diabetes."	
2. "I am old, gray, and disabled."	
3. "I can't decide. I will ask my children for their input."	
4. "I love my wife, and we have the best relationship."	
5. "I am very creative and productive in my daily work activities."	
6. "I know exactly who I am and where I am going."	
7. "I'm not sure that I can trust you with my timecard."	
8. "I have never been independent, and no one respects my feelings."	
9. "I have great feelings of self-reliance and adequacy."	
10. "You said that you still have strong feelings about not saying goodbye to your mother before she died?"	
11. "I went roller skating with my friend and never fell once."	
12. "I have a fragmented sense of self and feel inadequate most of the time."	
13. "You are so preoccupied with making money that you have neglected your family."	
14. "My overall attitude is good, and I am satisfied with my life."	
15. "I look forward to the day when I can retire."	
16. "I would rather work by myself than keep company with another."	

Answers to the Activity Related to Erikson's Eight Stages of Development

a. Mistrust	e. Inferiority	i. Shame	m. Identity
b. Autonomy	f. Integrity.	j. Isolation	n. Guilt
c. Intimacy	g. Self-absorption	k. Initiative	o. Industry
d. Despair	h. Identity diffusion	l. Generativity	p. Trust

Verbal Statements	Outcomes
1. "I will gladly be the spokesperson for diabetes."	Initiative
2. "I am old, gray, and disabled."	Despair
3. "I can't decide. I will ask my children for their input."	Inferiority
4. "I love my wife, and we have the best relationship."	Intimacy
5. "I am very creative and productive in my daily work activities."	Generativity
6. "I know exactly who I am and where I am going."	Identity
7. "I'm not sure that I can trust you with my timecard."	Mistrust
8. "I have never been independent, and no one respects my feelings."	Shame
9. "I have great feelings of self-reliance and adequacy."	Autonomy
10. "You said that you still have strong feelings about not saying goodbye to your mother before she died?"	Guilt
11. "I went roller skating with my friend and never fell once."	Industry
12. "I have a fragmented sense of self and feel inadequate most of the time."	Identity diffusion
13. "You are so preoccupied with making money that you have neglected your family."	Self-absorption
14. "My overall attitude is good, and I am satisfied with my life."	Trust
15. "I look forward to the day when I can retire."	Integrity
16. "I would rather work by myself than keep company with another."	Isolation

Psychoanalytic Theory

Freud's Psychosexual Theory

- Oral Stage—Birth–18 months

- Anal Stage—18 months–3 years

- Phallic Stage—3–6 years

- Oedipus Complex Stage—4–6 years

- Latency Stage—6–12 years

- Genital Stage—12–18 years

Erikson's Life Cycle Theory

- Trust versus Mistrust—0–2 Years

- Autonomy versus Shame/Doubt—2–4 Years

- Initiative versus Guilt—4–6 Years

- Industry versus Inferiority—6–12 years

- Identity versus Identity Diffusion—13–18 Years

- Intimacy versus Isolation—Young Adult

- Generativity versus Self-absorption—Middle Years

- Integrity versus Despair—Old Age

Piaget's Cognitive Theory of Development

- Sensorimotor—0–2 Years

- Preoperational—2–7 Years

- Concrete Operational—7–14 Years

- Formal Operations—14 Years–Adult

<u>Interpersonal Theory: Harry Stack Sullivan</u>

- Infancy—0–12 Months

- Childhood—1–6 Years

- Juvenile—6–9 Years

- Early Adolescence—9–12 Years

- Late Adolescence—12–18 Years

- Adulthood—18 Years

CHAPTER 5: The Biological Basis of Mental Illness

Case Presentation

Ms. L. is a 41-year-old client who is mildly retarded and who was diagnosed in her early 20s as having paranoid schizophrenia. She presented at the emergency room with intermittent torticollis and tremors of the upper extremities. According to her psychosocial history, which was verified through collaboration with family members, Ms. L. would alternate between acute psychotic episodes and remissions. Over a period of 20 years, she received numerous antipsychotic medications that cause neurologic side effects. The client's previous responses to the neuroleptic agents prescribed involved acute and chronic extrapyramidal side effects. The family reported that, after 10 years of receiving treatment of neuroleptic medications, she developed severe dyskinesia, which consisted of chewing movements, tongue motion, lip smacking, tongue protrusion ("fly catcher's tongue"), rapid eye blinking, cogwheel rigidity, and tremors in her lower extremities. These reactions caused the client great distress, and she became noncompliant with her medications. The selection of the medication was determined by the client's tolerance to side effects and was either changed to a newer antipsychotic medication or the dosage was reduced, which resulted in significant improvement in extrapyramidal symptoms.

Critical Thinking Issues

1. Discuss the various brain regions and their specific chemical messengers.

2. How do the functional or dysfunctional actions of the chemical messengers of the brain affect mental illness?

3. Discuss neurotransmitters and how neuroleptic agents play a major role.

4. What are the antipsychotic medications that block specific receptors of serotonin (the 5-HT_2) and dopamine (the D_2 receptors).

Student Activities

WORD-FIND PUZZLE

The following words are hidden in the puzzle. They may be read up or down, forward, backward, or diagonally, but always in a straight line. Some words may overlap, and some letters in the grid may be used more than once. Not all the letters in the grid will be used. Circle each word as your locate it.

ADAPTATION
ANTAGONIST
BASAL GANGLIA
BIOGENIC AMINES
BRAIN
CATECHOLAMINES
CEREBELLUM
CEREBRUM
CHOLINERGICS
CIRCADIAN RHYTHM
COGWHEEL
DIENCEPHALON
DYSTONIA

LIMBIC SYSTEM
LIP SMACKING
MEMBRANES
MENTAL ILLNESS
NEUROANATOMY
NEUROPEPTIDES
NEUROTRANSMITTERS
RELEASE
REMISSION
SCHIZOPHRENIA
SEROTONIN
STRESS

GENETICS
HEREDITY
HIPPOCAMPUS
HISTAMINE
HYPOTHALAMUS
IMMUNE
SYNAPSE
TARDIVE DYSKINESIA
THALAMUS
TONGUE MOTION
TORTICOLLIS
TREMORS

```
T S C W S N O I T O M E U G N O T C R D
O E A X E E N O I T A T P A D A I E A P
R N V S D U B R A I N U Y V R R A R I I
T A O S I R T I I X R T T D C E I E N N
I R H E T O R S O X E H I A T M N B E E
C B I N P T E T U G L V D T S I O E R U
O M P L E R M R D K E I I O I S T L H R
L E P L P A O E P D A N G F N S S L P O
L M O I O N R S Y N S E I F O I Y U O A
I E C L R S S R E E Y R C G O D M Z N
S T A A U M K H B A S A L G A N G L I A
C S M T E I Y T I D E R E H T M U K H T
C Y P N N T N O L A H P E C N E I D C O
R S U E H T S U M A L A H T A C G N S M
I C S M C E R E B R U M W I M M U N E Y
L I K S E R O T O N I N G E N E T I C S
A B D R F S E N I M A L O H C E T A C B
H M C H O L I N E R G I C S Y N A P S E
L I P S M A C K I N G H I S T A M I N E
A L C J B S U M L A H T O P Y H P P B N
```

37

PUZZLE SOLUTION

```
T S C W S N O I T O M E U G N O T C R D
O E A X E E N O I T A T P A D A I E A P
R N V S D U B R A I N U Y V R R A R I I
T A O S I R T I I X R T T D C E I E N N
I R H E T O R S O X E H I A T M N B E E
C B I N P T E T U G L V D T S I O E R U
O M P L E R M R D K E I I O I S T L H R
L E P L P A O E P D A N G F N S S L P O
L M O I O N R S Y N S E I F O I Y U O A
I E C L R S S R E E Y R C G O D M Z N
S T A A U M K H B A S A L G A N G L I A
C S M T E I Y T I D E R E H T M U K H T
C Y P N N T N O L A H P E C N E I D C O
R S U E H T S U M A L A H T A C G N S M
I C S M C E R E B R U M W I M M U N E Y
L I K S E R O T O N I N G E N E T I C S
A B D R F S E N I M A L O H C E T A C B
H M C H O L I N E R G I C S Y N A P S E
L I P S M A C K I N G H I S T A M I N E
A L C J B S U M L A H T O P Y H P P B N
```

38

Major Divisions of the Cortex

- Frontal Lobe

- Parietal Lobe

- Occipital Lobe

- Temporal Lobe

Neurotransmitters Involved in Psychiatric Illness

Biogenic Amines

- Catecholamines

  ▾ Indolamines

  ▾ Dopamine

  ▾ Norepinephrine

  ▾ Serotonin

  ▾ Histamine

- Cholinergics

  ▾ Acetylcholine

- Neuropeptides

- Amino Acids

CHAPTER 6: Psychopharmacology

Case Presentations

Suzie, a 15-year-old high school student, is escorted to the mental health center by her mother after a suicide attempt. During the initial assessment by the clinical nurse specialist (CNS), Suzie's mother reported that for the past 2 months her daughter had been very sad, withdrawn, unable to sleep, fatigued, and irritable at times. Her appetite was reduced, and she complained of feelings of hopelessness. Her school performance is lacking because of her impaired concentration and is of major concern. The only comment from Suzie was, "I just want get rid of these feelings." A prescription for fluoxetine was given to Suzie, and the dosage, frequency, and side effects were explained. Her mother listened attentively and then verbalized much concern about not wanting her daughter to take the medication because of the possibility that Suzie would become an addict. Suzie was discharged in the mother's care with an appointment in 1 week and with written instructions about the medication.

Critical Thinking Issues

1. How would you respond to the mother's concern?

2. Discuss the mother's feelings about addiction.

3. Discuss the mother-daughter relationship.

4. What factors helped to determine the CNS decision to prescribe fluoxetine?

5. What side effects should the CNS emphasize?

6. Discuss the importance of Suzie returning to the clinic in 1 week.

7. Discuss how the mother's attitude might influence Susie's compliance with taking fluoxetine.

Student Activities

JEOPARDY GAME WITH PSYCHOTROPIC MEDICINES

Answers on board under the following categories. Can be hidden by tabs, which say 100, 200, 300, 400, and 500. All questions are answered by either stating the drug or drug category to which the phrase is referring or by answering with the information, according to the category, about the drug on the board. Some answers can be starred,* and a bonus question can be asked. For example, under side effects, the answer, drooling and akinesia, merits the response, "What are antipsychotics?" Bonus points can be given for correctly naming the symptoms described, for example, pseudoparkinsonism.

MEDICATIONS

DRUG CATEGORIES	SIDE EFFECTS	PATIENT TEACHING	NURSING ACTIONS	GRAB BAG
A novel antidepressant	Agitation Insomnia gastro-intestinal distress	Report sore throat, fever	Monitor blood pressure	Used for narcolepsy
A novel antipsychotic	Divalproex	Blood drawn 10–12 hr after last dose	Monitor temperature	Mechanism of action for divalproex
Zolpidem	Drooling Akinesia	Avoid foods containing tyramine	Give benztropine	Target symptoms of risperidone
Ritalin	Priapism	Don't stop taking abruptly	Give with food	Psychostim. with least risk of dependency
Non-traditional anxiolytic	Appetite loss Insomnia	2–4 weeks to see effects	Treatment for akathisia	First symptoms relieved by antidepressants

ANSWERS CAN BE STATED IN QUESTION FORM

MEDICATIONS

DRUG CATEGORIES	SIDE EFFECTS	PATIENT TEACHING	NURSING ACTIONS	GRAB BAG
Any SSRI	SSRI Fluoxetine	Carbamazepine Clozapine—Blood dyscrasias	Orthostatic hypotension TCAs, MAOIs Antipsychotics	Psychostims
Clozapine Olanzapine Risperidone	Nausea, indigestion	Lithium	Clozapine and TCAs—blood dyscrasias Antipsychotics— NMS	Increase GABA
Ambien Sedative	Parkinsonism of antipsychotics	MAOIs	For EPS of antipsychotics	Positive and negative symptoms of schizophrenia
MAOI	Trazodone	Benzodiazepine and valproate increase risk of seizures	Lithium valproate to decrease GI distress	Pemoline
Buspirone Propanolol	Psychostim.	Antidepressant	Benzo- diazepines	Vegetative or physical symptoms

Extrapyramidal Syndrome

- Parkinsonism—tremors, drooling, shuffling gait, muscular rigidity

- Akathisia—restlessness

- Dystonia—muscle spasms of the jaw, tongue, neck, or eyes

- Akinesia—motor inertia

CHAPTER 7: Cognitive-Behavior Therapy

Case Presentation

Mr. K., a 37- year-old recently divorced man with one child, presented for treatment of overly aggressive and over-controlling behavior. He was unable to separate assertion and aggression. There appeared to be a loss of impulse control and appropriate problem solving. He revealed that there was a family history of physical abuse, violent outbursts, and alcohol abuse. He was one of four children and the only son. During the interview session, Mr. K. described himself as the athletic type who spent time lifting weights, muscle building, and exhibiting a high performance standard. He was proud of his masculinity. He felt pressured by his father to indulge in hard work and to be actively involved in community activities. Mr. K. stated that his father had a terrific temper that raged out of control, and he feared that he was following in his father's footsteps. In a torrent of words he stated, "I'm unaware of my anger until the situation builds and I have temper outbursts that are preceded by anxious feelings. I would go on a rampage, break dishes, and yell at my wife and child. I'm really a good moral person who lives by the rules, and I expect others to do the same. I'm an industrious, caring, and accommodating person, but I don't understand my behavior. I'm a perfectionist. I'm unaware of what I feel, so I find it difficult to get in touch with my feelings. I tried to live up to my father's expectations, but it never seemed to happen. I felt as though no one in my family loved me because they rarely spoke to me. My father was distant and involved only in his volunteer work. I've lost my wife; my family is distant; and I'm a complete failure. I know it is all my fault. I feel worthless and unworthy of help from any source." Mr. K. evaluates himself in a negative manner and berates himself for his rages.

Critical Thinking Issues

1. What effect has the environment had on the client's behavior?

2. What factors triggered the client's anger?

3. What behavioral technique can the nurse use?

4. Discuss the advantages of documenting the client's mood in a daily log.

5. Discuss the advantages of progressive relaxation.

Student Activities

Suggested Classroom Activity
In order to examine assertiveness among the classroom members, the students must be aware of the nonverbal messages being exhibited and their impact on others. Divide the class into pairs. Ask each participant to role play problematic interpersonal interactions and record the body language of his or her partner. Examine the emotions expressed verbally through reference to a body part. Identify the feeling message that is being conveyed.

Positive Body Signals	Body Response	Feeling Expressed
Smile		

Negative Body Signals	Body Response	Feeling Expressed
Poor Eye Contact		

Cognitive-Behavior Therapy

- Purpose

- Nurse's Role

- Behavioral Theories—Operant Conditioning

Procedures Used in Behavior Therapy

- Relaxation Exercises

- Biofeedback

- Desensitization

- Shaping

- Token Economics

- Extinction and Punishment

- Modeling

- Exposure-Response

- Social Skills Training

- Assertiveness Training

CHAPTER 8: Crisis Intervention

Case Presentation

Lilly, a 34-year-old woman who has a lengthy history of suicide attempts, was referred to the psychiatric hospital for admission because of a depressed mood and current suicidal ideation. A clinical nurse specialist interviewed Lilly and assessed her current problems and her family, marital, occupational, and mental health history. Specific emphasis was placed on her present suicidal ideation and on previous suicide attempts.

The interview revealed that the client's present suicide plan was to hang herself during the night while the rest of the family slept. Her first suicide attempt happened when she was 12 years old, and the other attempts happened every 7 years during periods when life was unbearablefor her. She stated that, "I was unable to cope with life any more." Three days prior to admission, the client experienced increased mood liability, poor concentration, decreased appetite, insomnia, and guilty ruminations. Other stressors that affected the balance of equilibrium for Lilly were social withdrawal and diminished interest in work activities. She described herself as having no close friends. She would like to be close to people but was fearful of rejection. She stated that she is "very sensitive to criticism and this plays an important role in her feelings toward people." She is self-critical and continues to have feelings of hopelessness and worthlessness. Further history revealed that she grew up in a physically and sexually abusive family. Her father sexually molested her between the ages of 8 and 14 years. Lilly's mother committed suicide when Lilly was 10 years old, and Lilly has blamed herself stating that, "If I had been a better child maybe this would never have happened." Lilly was involved in two abusive marriages and has two children from the first union. The teenagers, a daughter and a son, are living at home and, according to the client, are very supportive. However, the daughter will be leaving for college shortly, and Lilly feels anxious and ambivalent about her departure. The nurse explained that when a member of the family leaves, there is a major adjustment to make. Lilly began to cry and stated that she realizes the house will be empty without her daughter. She is also concerned that her present husband will leave her because she perceives herself as a burden. Lilly is currently employed as a pharmacist's assistant and has been employed with the same company for 10 years, even though she has had several episodes of depression. She is fearful that her employer will terminate her employment this time. She said "I don't know what I will do. We need the money because my husband doesn't make enough to support the household."

Critical Thinking Issues

1. Discuss the events that precipitated the client's crisis.

2. What upset in the state of emotional equilibrium has Lilly experienced?

3. What phase of the crisis state is Lilly experiencing?

4. What nursing interventions would be most helpful in the state of disequilibrium?

5. What are the collaborate problems that need to be addressed?

Student Activities

1. The four-phase paradigm of a crisis is listed below. Match the phases with the statements that describe the phases.
   a. Phase one
   b. Phase two
   c. Phase three
   d. Phase four

The individual's anxiety continues to rise, and the increased tension moves the individual to reach out for assistance and use every available resource to solve the problem and reduce the increasingly painful state of anxiety.

Answer: Phase three

The individual's response to a traumatic event causes an increase in the level of anxiety. The individual responds with the usual coping mechanisms in an attempt to reduce or eliminate the stress and discomfort arising from the excessive anxiety.

Answer: Phase one

If the individual's usual coping skills fail, he or she becomes more anxious, causing the initial rise in tension to continue.

Answer: Phase two

The state of active crisis results when internal strength and social support systems are inadequate, the problem remains unresolved, and tension and anxiety rise to an intolerable degree.

Answer: Phase four

2. As a volunteer service to the community, have students offer their services to the crisis intervention center. These centers are staffed by clinicians and volunteers.

3. In small groups, encourage students to share their stressful experiences and to discuss their perception of the event, support system, coping strategies, and resolution of the problem.

Directions: Listed below are situations that may precipitate a crisis state. After reading each event, determine whether each situation illustrates a developmental, situational, sociocultural, or adventitious crisis.

SITUATION	CRISIS			
	Developmental	**Sociocultural**	**Adventitious**	**Situation**
1. The town witnesses a mass murder.	☐	☐	☐	☐
2. A mother has terminal cancer.	☐	☐	☐	☐
3. A tornado demolished the Gulf Coast.	☐	☐	☐	☐
4. Mary experienced a sexual assault.	☐	☐	☐	☐
5. J. witnessed his father's murder.	☐	☐	☐	☐
6. G. retired after 57 years of work.	☐	☐	☐	☐
7. S. gave birth to her first child.	☐	☐	☐	☐
8. The young person married.	☐	☐	☐	☐
9. J. graduated from college.	☐	☐	☐	☐
10. People were displaced during urban upgrading.	☐	☐	☐	☐
11. Several banks were robbed recently.	☐	☐	☐	☐
12. Discriminatory practice caused J. to lose his job.	☐	☐	☐	☐
13. A. is wheelchair bound.	☐	☐	☐	☐
14. Women are valueless.	☐	☐	☐	☐
15. J. lost his executive position through downsizing.	☐	☐	☐	☐
16. J. feels he is "too old" and "useless."	☐	☐	☐	☐

Types of Crises

- Situational

- Maturational

- Adventitious

- Sociocultural

<u>Stages of Crisis Intervention</u>

- Assessment

- Determination of Scope

- Impact of the Crisis Experience

- Planning Therapeutic Intervention

- Intervention

- Resolution

- Anticipatory Planning

Methods of Crisis Intervention

- Generic Approach

- Environmental Manipulation

- Anticipatory Intervention

- Individual Approach

- Therapeutic Techniques

- Pharmacologic Intervention

CHAPTER 9: Group Therapy and Therapeutic Groups

Case Presentation

You have been asked to start an inpatient group for the following patients.

Jim, 35: Diagnosed with chronic paranoid schizophrenia; admitted 2 days ago; admitted with auditory hallucinations.

Sam, 67: Diagnosed with major depression, recurrent; admitted with psychomotor agitation 3 days ago.

Bev, 40: Diagnosed with bipolar disorder; admitted 2 days ago with symptoms of grandiose delusions, psychomotor agitation, flight of ideas, and insomnia for 3 days.

Susan, 37: Admitted 2 days ago with diagnosis of dysthymia with suicidal ideation but no plan.

Jean, 29: Diagnosed with major depression secondary to substance abuse, admitted 3 days ago with sleep disturbance, anhedonia, anergic, lack of appetite, and profound hopelessness.

Mike, 62: Retired steelworker who has been depressed since retirement on disability following an accident that caused head trauma.

Richard, 35: Diagnosed with schizophrenia, undifferentiated type, readmitted today because of noncompliance with medications.

Ann, 75: Admitted today with a diagnosis of dementia and has a hearing impairment

Jim, 55: Unemployed mechanic, admitted 5 days ago for detoxification with a diagnosis of substance abuse; ETOH is the drug of choice.

Sarah, 93: Diagnosed with Alzheimer's disease; admitted 3 days ago with loud persistent disorganized speech and picking in the air.

Critical Thinking Issues

1. List, with rationale, several types of groups that would be appropriate for these patients.

2. Choose one of the groups you have identified and identify which therapeutic factors might be evident with this type of group. Justify your selection.

3. What problems might you anticipate with this group process?

4. What leader functions are necessary so that the group is most likely to be effective?

5. If you had the opportunity to restructure this group (e..g., remove members, divide into two groups), which members would you remove from the group? Discuss your decision.

6. How would you evaluate the group's effectiveness?

Student Activities

Group Activity

DISCUSSION QUESTIONS: Within your classroom setting or clinical group, discuss your answers to the following questions.

1. Describe the group leader's responsibility for membership selection, providing for a physical setting that is conducive to an effective group meeting and preparing the client for the group.

2. Define co-leadership. Discuss when co-leadership of a group is beneficial. What problems might be anticipated when groups have co-leaders? What must occur for co-leaders to work effectively together?

3. Compare and contrast the use of group intervention strategies by the group leader.

4. Define group norms. Describe, with rationale, which norms should be identified by the leader from the beginning of the group and reinforced as the group continues to meet.

5. Discuss the role of the nurse in group therapy. Describe, with rationale, the areas of group therapy that need further research.

Therapeutic Factors

- Instillation of Hope

- Universality

- Imparting Information

- Altruism

- Corrective Recapitulation of the Primary Family Group

- Development of Socializing Techniques

- Imitative Behaviors

- Interpersonal Learning

- Group Cohesiveness

- Catharsis

- Existential Factors

- Group Purpose

- Goals

- Nurse's Role

- Membership Selection

- Group Environment

- Client Preparation

Stages of Group Development

- Initial Phase

- Responsive Phase

- Focused Phase

- Termination Phase

CHAPTER 10: Family Therapy

Case Presentation

The Casey family lives in a Southern rural town. Stella is a 27-year-old single mother of three children (Andrew age 10, Kim age 7, and Frank age 3 months). Her husband left the family soon after her mother died. She lives with her father, Luke, who is 50 years of age. Her mother died at the age of 49 of a massive heart attack. Luke is the active breadwinner of the family. Stella is the third of five siblings (Jimmy age 30, Kim age 28, Martha age 22, and Anthony age 19). All of the adults are active functioning adults in the community. Anthony is the only sibling who is pursuing a college education. The family is emotionally very close. The family does not put much emphasis on health promotion and emotional consulting. They only seek medical attention on rare occasions when sick.

Stella began to avoid her family members and showed no joy or spontaneity. Her family members became concerned when she showed no interest in caring for her children and the home environment. An appointment was made with a family nurse psychotherapist.

Critical Thinking Issues

1. Identify relevant assessment data from the information given in the case study.

2. What family health assessment tool(s) could the nurse use to identify the need(s) of this family?

3. What are the two priority NANDA (nursing diagnoses) for the family as a unit of care?

4. Describe some family nursing interventions for assisting the client with the two nursing diagnoses identified.

5. Describe relevant outcome criteria for evaluating nursing care for the client and the client's family.

6. Using a selected family system, identify the boundaries of the Casey family-of-origin data.

7. Apply the family life cycle development of Stella's nuclear family structure.

8. How many generations can you assess in the case study?

9. How would you approach the family membership in the case study?

10. Give an example of the emotional ties in the case study.

11. In which ways do you consider the family above as a "troubled" family?

Student Activities

Classroom Activity

Each student will have 45 minutes in class time, or overnight if preferred, to prepare the assigned case study and several minutes to report the content to the class. This activity will work well in a group format.

Each student will complete a structural mapping family process (review content in Figure 10–2 in your textbook) of the Casey family case study. Include in the assignment each of the following:

1. Identify the primary client.

2. List the identifying characteristics of each family member.

3. Given the information in Chapter 10, brainstorm about possible methods of meeting the needs of the Casey family.

4. Using NANDA (nursing diagnoses), write a nursing care study for the assigned family case study.

Family Therapy

- Purpose

- Nurse's Role

- Assessing the Family System

  ▾ Genogram

  ▾ Structural Mapping

- Family Assessment Guide

  ▾ Demographic Factors

  ▾ Sociocultural Factors

  ▾ Historical Factors

  ▾ Developmental Factors

  ▾ Development of Children

  ▾ Couple Development

  ▾ Family Life Cycle Development

Transparency

- Transactional Factors

  ▾ Communication

  ▾ Roles

  ▾ Boundaries

  ▾ Power

  ▾ Problem Solving

  ▾ Affective Factors

  ▾ Trust

  ▾ Mood and Tone

  ▾ Meanings

  ▾ Relational Integrity

Family Therapy Approaches

- Multigenerational Theories

- Bowen's Family System Theory

- Contextual Family Therapy

- Object Relations Theory

- Structural Family Therapy

- Systematic Family Therapy

- Psychoeducational Approach

CHAPTER 11: Sexual Therapy

Case Presentation

Mr. B., a 40-year-old corporate executive, sought therapy for treatment of erectile dysfunction. He stated that his marriage has been a disappointment and he has engaged in many extramarital affairs. During the assessment, he revealed that the reason for his infidelity was poor sex and a nagging wife. He stated that the first affair began when he hired an attractive secretary who was also in a bad marriage. He described their relationship as extremely passionate, a whirlwind affair, and thought that he had found the love of his life. He was immensely attracted to and obsessively preoccupied with this woman. A decision was made to begin living together, but subsequently she terminated her employment and quickly moved out of state with another man, leaving no forwarding address. Mr. B. was emotionally devastated. He spent long hours fantasizing about her and masturbating. He became involved in several one-night stands, but no one was as satisfying as the first affair. His attempts to function sexually were difficult and often unsuccessful, and he could not feel the sexual interest in any of the other women. Mr. B. is concerned about his libido and the possibility of becoming permanently impotent.

Critical Thinking Issues

1. What factors have influenced Mr. B.'s sexual behavior?

2. Discuss the cause of Mr. B.'s erectile dysfunction.

3. If Mr. B. was referred for sexual therapy, what areas should the therapist address?

4. Discuss the goal of treatment.

Student Activities

Classroom Activity

Interview a peer using the Guidelines for Sexual Interview (Table 11–2) in the *Contemporary Psychiatric–Mental Health Nursing* text.

1. Analyze your reaction to the interview, and compare it with the Possible Nurses' Reaction in Table 11–1.

2. Discuss the medications that may alter sexual behavior.

3. If possible, interview a client who is suffering from a sexual dysfunction.

4. Organize the data and develop a logical solution to the problem.

Sexual Therapy

- Purpose

- Nurse's Role

- Assessment of Sexual Functioning

- Referral for Sexual Therapy

Sexual Therapy Models

- Cognitive–Behavioral

- Psychodynamic and Psychosexual

- Systems

CHAPTER 12: Reminiscence Therapy

Case Presentation

Jane, a 79-year-old African-American woman, became increasingly depressed after being admitted to a local nursing home. She was diagnosed with her third cardiovascular accident. There was no one to care for her in her home. She has two adult children, both of whom live out of town. She was in no condition to travel. Jane would only communicate with the staff by crying out, "You are hurting me." Jane would only communicate by responding to yes/no questions. The nurse diagnosed Jane with selective aphasia. Her son and her friends were very attentive during the course of the admission process. The family and friends' visits soon decreased.

The staff nurse continued to monitor Jane's mental status. She decided that because of Jane's continued isolation and depressive symptoms, she needed some type of intervention. The intervention of choice was a reminiscence group. The group met every Thursday morning. Jane continued to be silent and did not share in the group's discussion. The nurse noted that even though Jane was silent, she was attentive and appeared to be listening. The nurse talked with Jane's son about her hobbies, life's work, and other interests. Jane loved to shop and travel. She was always conscious of weight gain. Jane also loved watching football , the news reports, and daytime soap operas.

The reminiscence group members began talking about their life's work and experiences with peers and bosses. Jane contributed to the group and made jokes about her formal job-related tasks. Jane continued to participate in the group discussion and hated to miss the group members when she was not able to participate in the session. In the unit, Jane interacted with the members of the group and her family when they visited.

Critical Thinking Issues

1. Identify relevant assessment data from the information given in the case study that showed that Jane would benefit from participating in reminiscence group therapy sessions.

2. Given the information available to you, state identified familial influences that contributed to Jane's care.

   - Positive Influences:

   - Negative Influences:

3. Write a NANDA (nursing diagnosis) for Jane's plan of care.

4. List identifying characteristics of a reminiscence group therapy session.

5. What are the needs of the group members in a life review group session?

6. Define techniques for assessing clients who are in need of reminiscence therapy.

7. Distinguish between simple and informative reminiscence therapy and life review.

8. Discuss appropriate use of reminiscence therapy.

9. How might the staff nurse go about influencing a client that group intervention would be an asset to his or her care?

10. Discuss how you would evaluate the outcomes of a reminiscence therapy group.

Student Activities

Objectives:

1. To conduct a student-oriented group process activity using reminiscence as a main focus as evidenced by the students embellishing on a perfect day activity.

2. Explain the appropriate nursing care in relation to reminiscence as an appropriate nursing intervention as evidenced by discussing the nurse's role in reminiscence therapy.

3. Using your textbook (see Chapter 12), apply current research findings to selected intervention concepts for reminiscence therapy.

Using the "perfect day activity" attached, ask the students to form a mock activity group.

Each student group will:

1. Participate in the group process.

2. Use a process-oriented format by choosing a leader, scribe, reporter, and evaluator.

3. Follow the directions on the assignment sheet.

Each student will have 45 minutes to participate in a mock reminiscence therapy group. The reporter will share with the entire class the process and effectiveness of reminiscence as a therapy intervention. The evaluator will share with the class the outcome of the group members' effectiveness as a working group.

The Perfect Day Activity

Goal: To share with the group members my life activities during a perfect day.

Procedure:

1. The leader of the group is to list the following questions on newsprint or chalkboard and ask that the group members respond to them as indicated.

2. The members of the group are to share the information with their peers.

3. The scribe will share information with the group regarding reminiscence therapy and its effectiveness as a nursing intervention.

4. The evaluator will share with the members of the class the effectiveness of the members as a working group.

Questions:

1. What elements of your perfect day were absolutely indispensable to your up bringing?

2. Remembering back to your upbringing, where would you spend your perfect day?

3. Close your eyes, and imagine a perfect day. What feelings do you get during your perfect day?

4. What elements of your ideal perfect day do you have with you in the present?

5. Use the following scale from 1 to 10, and check where your ideal perfect day would be measured.

    −   +

1 _____ **10**

Types of Reminiscence

- Simple

- Informative

- Life Review

- Oral History

- Autobiography

Definition of Reminiscence Therapy

- Use of Simple and Informational Reminiscence as a Nursing Intervention for Treatment of Specific Psychosocial Nursing Diagnoses

- Purposes of Reminiscence Therapy

- Nurse's Role

CHAPTER 13: Milieu Therapy

Case Presentation

Paul is a 34-year-old single man who lives at home with his widowed mother. He is diagnosed as:

I—Bipolar Disorder, most recent episode manic

II—None

III—Malnutrition

He has been in and out of psychiatric hospitals since the age of 21. This is his sixth hospitalization. His symptomatology has been adequately controlled with lithium. He usually stabilizes quickly and is discharged. However, after several months, he stops taking his medication and within weeks he has a relapse. Prior to admission, he was not sleeping or eating. He has lost 14 lb. His grooming and hygiene were poor. He claims that he has made a fantastic business deal and is rich. Upon admission, he paced constantly, talked loudly, and was unable to sleep. He also refused to bathe and would not sit to eat. He doesn't think that he needs to be in the hospital and insists that he must leave to finish his business deal. He is intrusive and uses other clients' belongings.

Critical Thinking Issues

1. Assess Paul's nursing needs and identify nursing interventions to address Gunderson's five milieu functions:

   Containment

   Support

   Structure

   Involvement

   Validation

2. What function would be the initial priority, and why?

3. What "unacceptable" behaviors would require limit setting?

4. Identify expected outcomes of care.

5. How can staff behavior adversely affect client recovery?

6. What staff behaviors promote a trusting atmosphere?

7. What information should be provided to a client during orientation?

8. How does a thorough orientation help to promote a therapeutic milieu?

9. Why is an attitude of permissiveness, in which there is tolerance of all behavior, counterproductive to a therapeutic milieu?

10. Discuss how a client's rights and decreased length of stay influenced the shift from therapist-focused individual therapy to multidisciplinary, milieu therapy.

11. Discuss the advantages of group process over individual therapy.

12. How would you structure a daily schedule from wake-up to bedtime that ensures a high level of interaction between clients and staff?

13. In what other settings could milieu management principles be applied?

Student Activities

WORD PUZZLE

Insert the following key terms into the word puzzle below.

Orientation   Containment   Empathy
Group   Nurturance   Schedule
Structure   Involvement   Support
Individuality   Communication
Validation   Multidisciplinary

```
_  _ _ _ _ _  _ M _ _ _
   _ _ _ _ _ _ I _ _ _
     _ _ L _ _ _ _ _ _
     _ _ I _ _ _ _ _ _ _ _
       _ _ _ E _ _ _ _
         _ _ U _ _ _ _ _

   _ _ _ _ T _ _
   _ _ _ _ _ H _
   _ _ _ _ _ _ E _ _ _ _
       _ _ _ R _ _ _ _
     _ _ _ _ _ _ A _ _ _ _
         _ _ _ _ P _ _ _
   _ _ _ _ _ _ _ _ _ _ _ Y
```

Key for Word Puzzle

1. Containment
2. Multidisciplinary
3. Validation
4. Orientation
5. Schedule
6. Support
7. Structure
8. Empathy
9. Involvement
10. Nurturance
11. Communication
12. Group
13. Individuality

Milieu Therapy

- Purpose

- Functions

  - ▾ Containment

  - ▾ Support

  - ▾ Structure

  - ▾ Involvement

  - ▾ Validation

- Nurse's Role as Milieu Manager

CHAPTER 14: Electroconvulsive Therapy and Other Biological Therapies

Case Presentation

Ms. W. is a 65-year-old retiree with a history of depression. She has been married for 40 years to her childhood sweetheart, who has always been very supportive. Ms. W.'s husband became concerned when he noticed that his wife refused to eat and showed self-neglect, which, he claimed, "was highly unusual for her." During the interview, Ms. W. tells the nurse that retirement was not as she expected and she is very depressed. Her husband was present during the initial assessment process and reported that his wife had been hospitalized a number of times for major depression. She was given numerous antidepressant medications for recurrent depression, and she had received two electroconvulsive therapy (ECT) treatments. He also revealed that her depressive illness episodes included suicide attempts.

Nursing assessment revealed that the client is severely depressed, has difficulty concentrating, exhibits feelings of hopelessness and worthlessness, and is unable to acknowledge her personal achievements and attributes. She is pessimistic about the future and her ability to accept her retiree status. She states that she feels inadequate, apathetic, and lacks motivation. Ms. W. states that, "God is her salvation and she will meet her maker very soon." Ms. W. is a well-nourished, slightly overweight person who appears to be in good physical health. The client's blood pressure is 150/90 mm Hg; pulse rate is 96 beats/min; and respirations are 22 breaths/min.

Ms. W. was admitted to the psychiatric unit, and it was determined by the interdisciplinary team that she should receive ECT. When Ms. W. was informed about the pending ECT treatments, she expressed fear and anxiety. Her main concern was loss of memory and how soon it would return.

The ECT procedure was explained to Ms. W., and she was informed that it would be necessary for her to sign a consent form because ECT requires administration of anesthesia.

Critical Thinking Issues

1. Discuss the significant factors that would indicate the necessity of ECT.

2. Discuss informed consent and the State statues that relate to ECT.

3. How can the nurse help Ms. W. and her family deal with the fear of ECT treatments?

4. Develop a teaching plan to help prepare the client for ECT?

5. ECT is a vital component of the treatment plan for clients with mood disturbance. Analyze this statement.

Student Activities

It is necessary to exhibit caution when electroconvulsive therapy (ECT) is administered to clients with intracranial pressure, clients who are pregnant, and those who have had a recent myocardial infarction. How can the nurse provide a safe environment?

1. Identify the risk factors.

2. Utilizing the nursing process, design a plan of care for one of the aforementioned conditions.

3. Informed consent is a vital component when helping a client choose the procedure. List the nursing considerations useful in ensuring that the client understands the treatment and the implications.

4. Describe the importance of documentation of the informed consent.

5. Describe the legal implications related to ETC.

6. Identify two nursing measures related to the expected outcome. The client will have resolution of behaviors associated with severe depression.

7. Identify two nursing measures related to the expected outcome. The client will have improved quality of life.

Electroconvulsive Therapy

- Theory of Action

- Indications

- Contraindictations

- Risk Factors

- Adverse Effects

Electroconvulsive Therapy (ECT)

Conditions for which ECT may be beneficial:

- Severe major depression

- Severe major depression with psychotic features

- Bipolar disorder (manic, depressed, or mixed phases)

- Severe mood disorder during pregnancy

- Major depression in older adults

- Schizophrenia, particularly with catatonic or affective symptoms

- Postpartum psychosis

CHAPTER 15: Delirium, Dementia, and Amnestic and Other Disorders

Case Presentation

A physically strong and previously independent elderly man, who was in the fourth stage of Alzheimer's disease, was relocated to his daughter's household because of financial problems. This placed a severe financial burden and an intense psychological and physical stress on the daughter. Within 9 months and following a Global Deterioration Scale (GDS) assessment by his physician, the client's daughter was told that her father was now in the fifth stage.

Critical Thinking Issues

1. What behaviors are commonly found in the fourth stage?

2. What additional changes in his behavior can be expected as a result of this environmental change?

3. What home adjustments will his daughter have to make in order to provide a safe setting?

4. What groups are available to provide support for the daughter?

5. What are the clinical characteristics associated with the fifth stage of Alzheimer's disease?

6. As her father experiences an additional cognitive decline, associated with the fifth stage, what other changes will the daughter have to make in order to adequately provide for her father's physical, psychological, spiritual, and safety needs?

Case Presentation

The nurse observes that a 75-year-old nursing home resident, whose diagnosis is dementia, has night wandering episodes called sundowning.

Critical Thinking Issues

1. What are the common symptoms of sundowning?

2. What nursing care should be planned and provided for the client who experiences this problem?

3. In the twentyfirst century, what economic, technologic, and sociocultural trends will have the greatest impact on Americans suffering from dementing illness?

Student Activities

Cross-Word Puzzle

Dementia versus Depression

Directions:

1. Read the clue and identify the word.
2. Write the appropriate missing word in the blank space of the sentence.
3. Print the word in the numbered space on the puzzle grid.

<u>Across</u> (Dementia)

<u>Clue</u>

6. Inclination to hesitate.
   <u>Sentence</u>: _____ in mood and behavior is common.
7. Extending upward relatively little.
   <u>Sentence</u>: Suicide risk in later stages of the disorder is _____.
9. To conceal.
   <u>Sentence</u>: Attempts are made by this client to _____ deficits.
10. Having a more serious effect than is apparent.
    <u>Sentence</u>: The onset of this disorder is_____.
12. Faulty or inaccurate.
    <u>Sentence</u>: The client with this disorder usually answers questions_____.
13. Apart from others.
    <u>Sentence</u>: This client often feels _____during the beginning stage of the illness.
15. A condition of deteriorated mentality.
    <u>Sentence</u>: _____is a chronic irreversible change in structure and function of the brain.
16. Lasting; firmly established.
    <u>Sentence</u>: Cognitive impairment is comparably_____during the beginning stage, with a steady worsening over the years.
18. Manifest; noticeable.
    <u>Sentence</u>: Symptoms of sundown syndrome are more _____during the evening hours, when there is less light and environmental stimuli.
19. Not brief; too long.
    <u>Sentence</u>: Symptoms are present for a _____period of time.
20. To hide or withdraw from observation.
    <u>Sentence</u>: This client often attempts to_____memory gaps during interactions.
21. Rare; infrequent.
    <u>Sentence</u>: A history of psychiatric disturbance is usually_____for this client.

Down (Depression)

<u>Clue</u>

1. Happening at short intervals; often repeated.
   <u>Sentence</u>: past disturbances in the depressed client's psychiatric history are usually_____.
2. The official mark stamped on articles to attest their purity.
   <u>Sentence</u>: Fatigue and lethargy are _____symptoms of this disorder.
3. Elevated ; lofty.
   <u>Sentence</u>: Risk for suicide can be_____.
4. Excitement of feeling, accompanied by attention and concern.
   <u>Sentence</u>: Lack of _____is often evident when the client responds, "I don't know."
5. Continually occurring
   <u>Sentence</u>: Depressed mood is usually_____until the client responds to therapy.
8. To emphasize or make prominent in various ways.
   <u>Sentence</u>: During this illness, deficits and disabilities are_____.
11. Dejection, as of mind.
    <u>Sentence</u>: The discovery of _____is an abnormal extension, or overelaboration, of sadness and grief.
14. To make a difference, or change from one another.
    <u>Sentence</u>: Cognitive impairments may_____ greatly in the depressed client.
17. Swift; rapid.
    <u>Sentence</u>: this disorder often has a_____onset.

THERAPEUTIC NURSE–PATIENT COMMUNICATION GRID

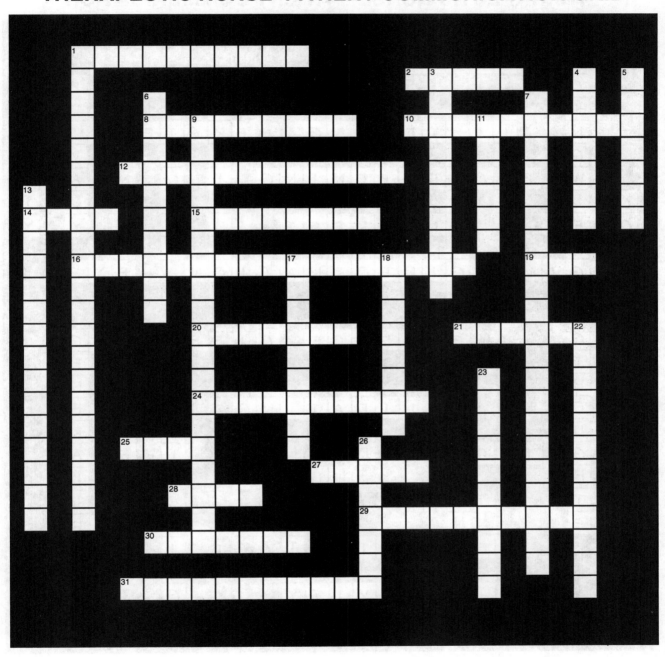

THERAPEUTIC NURSE–PATIENT COMMUNICATION

Across

1. ACCEPTANCE
2. SPACE
8. LISTENING
10. PROTECTION
12. BROADOPENING
14. OPEN
15. INTEREST
16. GIVINGINFORMATION
19. EYE
20. SILENCE
21. FACING
24. VALIDATING
25. TACT
27. HUMOR
28. TONE
29. ASSISTANCE
30. RESPECT
31. OBJECTIVITY

Down

1. ACKNOWLEDGING
3. SEMISSION
4. PR
5. HONESTY
6. CLARIFYING
7. ACKNOWLEDGING
9. SHARING
11. TIMING
13. CONFIDENTIALITY
17. OPENENDED
18. TOUCHING
22. GENERALLEADS
23. REFLECTING
26. EMPATH

Delirium

- Result of an Underlying Medical Condition

- Substance Induced

- Substance Withdrawal

Dementia

- Alzheimer's Type

- Vascular Dementia

- Dementia Due to Head Trauma

- Substance-Induced Dementia

- Dementia Due to Human Immunodeficiency Virus(HIV)

- Dementia Due to Parkinson's Disease

- Dementia Due to Huntington's Disease

- Dementia Due to Pick's Disease

CHAPTER 16: Mental Illness Due to a General Medical Condition

Case Presentation

Ms. C., a 30-year-old with recent psychotic episodes and a history of hyperthyroidism, was not taking medication when she was admitted for treatment. Her family reported that she experiences restlessness, excitability, agitation, and emotional instability. On evaluation, Ms. C. stated that she feels insecure and anxious, and she has become dependent on family members. She explained that she is extremely sensitive and fears rejection. Ms. C. is concerned about her physical health because of excessive weight loss during the past 6 months despite her increased appetite. She feels weak and fatigued and suffers from heat intolerance, diarrhea, and insomnia. During the interview, the nurse observed that the client exhibited fine tremors of the hands.

Critical Thinking Issues

1. List a nursing diagnosis related to this situation.

2. What is the most important nursing intervention for this client?

3. State an expected outcome related to each nursing diagnosis.

4. What is the interface between biology and behavior with regard to hyperthyroidism?

Student Activities

Fill in the blanks:

1. Characteristic behaviors and early signs of mental illness due to a general medical condition may include_____, _____, _____ or _____, and _____.

2. Visual hallucinations may be an indicator of exposure to some _____.

3. During their hospital stay,_____percent of persons older than 65 years of age develop_____.

4. Hyperthyroidism is known to cause psychiatric problems such as _____ and _____.

5. Initial psychiatric symptoms related to hyperthroidism often include_____, _____, _____, and _____.

6. Head trauma can bring on a variety of mental changes. Initial symptoms may include _____and_____.

7. The client with head trauma may experience_____and_____responses related to confusion and amnesia.

8. Chronic neurologic conditions such as _____and_____are associated with psychiatric symptoms.

9. Nursing interventions for the hospitalized client need to be focused on_____, _____, and_____,_____, and _____.

10. Nursing interventions for the client who is agitated, combative, or hostile should be directed at providing a _____,_____,and_____.

11. Critical care unit (CCU) psychosis is often_____and_____.

12. Planning care for the client with mental illness due to a general medical condition may be difficult for the unprepared staff because they sometimes _____the_____ or_____until they become_____.

94

Answers

1. Characteristic behaviors and early signs of mental illness due to a general medical condition may include <u>angry outbursts</u>, <u>anxiety</u>, <u>euphoria</u> or <u>depression</u>, and <u>disinhibitions</u>.

2. Visual hallucinations may be an indicator of exposure to some <u>toxic substance</u>.

3. During their hospital stay, <u>10 to 15</u>% of persons older than 65 years of age develop <u>delirium</u>.

4. Hyperthyroidism is known to cause psychiatric problems such as <u>phobias</u> and <u>manic behavior</u>.

5. Initial psychiatric symptoms related to hyperthyroidism often include <u>sleeplessness</u>, <u>anxiety</u>, <u>emotional lability</u>, and <u>difficulty concentrating</u>.

6. Head trauma can bring on a variety of mental changes. Initial symptoms may include <u>confusion</u> and <u>amnesia</u>.

7. The client with head trauma may experience <u>anxiety</u> and phobic responses related to confusion and amnesia.

8. Chronic neurologic conditions such as <u>multiple sclerosis</u> and <u>Parkinson's disease</u> are associated with psychiatric symptoms.

9. Nursing interventions for the hospitalized client need to be focused on <u>physical assessment</u>, <u>monitoring vital signs</u>, and <u>maintenance of fluid and nutrition intake</u>, <u>sleep-wake cycle</u>, and <u>skin</u> <u>care</u>.

10. Nursing interventions for the client who is agitated, combative, or hostile should be directed at providing a <u>calm</u>, <u>safe environment</u> and <u>setting limits</u>.

11. Critical care unit (CCU) psychosis is often <u>unrecognized</u> and <u>poorly diagnosed</u>.

12. Planning care for the client with mental illness due to a general medical condition may be difficult for the unprepared staff because they sometimes <u>overlook</u> the <u>symptoms</u> or <u>avoid dealing with them</u> until they become <u>extreme</u>.

Common Mental Illnesses That May Be Due to General Medical Conditions

- Delirium

- Dementia

- Amnestic Disorder

- Psychotic Disorder

- Mood Disorder

- Anxiety Disorder

- Sleep Disorder

- Personality Change

- Catatonia

- Mental Disorder Not Otherwise Specified

CHAPTER 17: Substance-Related Disorders

Case Presentation

Stanley is a 40-year-old divorced, homeless, and unemployed man who is currently in a day treatment program. He has been using heroin for the past 20 years and has made many attempts to stop using this substance. He has been a client in numerous treatment facilities and programs. He has also tried various self-help groups. His family has grown weary of his addiction and numerous failed attempts at sobriety. They feel that they have spent a lot of money on him and lost a great deal due to the amount he has stolen from them. Stanley states that this time will be different and that he has learned his lesson. He was referred to the methadone clinic and was provided with the drug. He has attended all of the scheduled meetings and is looking forward to a healthier mental and physical state of well-being.

Critical Thinking Issues

1. Discuss the substitution of methadone for heroin.

2. What criteria might the nurse use to determine if a client is serious about treatment?

3. Discuss the positive outcomes of his behavior.

4. What other community resources may be available for Stanley?

Student Activities

Unscramble the following words related to substance-related disorders.

1. heapruio   _____

2. lfuisriamd   _____

3. etconlaer   _____

4. annigebl   _____

5. inaccoe   _____

6. ledain   _____

7. sngtatioan   _____

8. lwevet etpss   _____

9. smearf   _____

10. srach   _____

11. ateoenlrxn   _____

12. lath   _____

Answers

1.	heapruio	euphoria
2.	lfuisriamd	disulfiram
3.	etconlaer	tolerance
4.	annigebl	enabling
5.	inaccoe	cocaine
6.	ledain	denial
7.	sngtatioan	antagonist
8.	lwevet etpss	twelve steps
9.	smearf	frames
10.	srach	crash
11.	ateoenlrxn	naltexone
12.	lath	halt

Substance-Related Disorder

Definition

Characteristic Behaviors

- Substance Abuse

- Alcohol Abuse

- Substance Dependence

- Enabling

- Intoxication and Withdrawal

Culture, Age, and Gender Features

- Culture

- Age

- Gender

Etiology

- Biological Theories

- Imaging Studies

- Genetic Theories

- Behavioral Theories

Prognosis

Assessment

- Short Alcohol and Drug History

- Screening Tools

- Family and Significant Others

- Physical Findings and Mental Status Examination

- Laboratory Findings

Planning Care

Intervention for Hospitalized Clients

- Acute Intoxication

- Acute Withdrawal

Interventions for Clients in the Community

- Brief Interventions

- Cognitive-Behavior Therapy

- Long-Term Substance Dependence

- Family Interventions

- Pharmacologic Treatments

- Alcohol and Opioid Dependence

- Benzodiazepines and Sedative-Hypnotic Withdrawal

- Stimulant Withdrawal

- Nicotine Withdrawal

Expected Outcomes

Differential Diagnosis

- Medical Disorders

- Mood Disorders

- Psychotic Disorders

- Anxiety Disorders

CHAPTER 18: Schizophrenia and Other Psychotic Disorders

Case Presentation

A 23-year-old African American single male who was diagnosed as having schizophrenia paranoid type presented at the community mental health clinic complaining of auditory hallucinations. The client was reevaluated for medication compliance and a possible change in medication regimen. During the mental status assessment, the clinical nurse specialist observed that the client was poorly groomed, had periods of agitation, and exhibited several explosive outbursts. His behavior had changed recently as he had become irritable and expressed more overt anger. The client stated that he was going through living arrangement changes that were stressful and caused intense anxiety. He expressed delusions of reference and prejudice and spoke of racial conspiracy. He heard people talking about him. The voices consisted of insulting comments on his behavior, which the client contributed to members of the temporary living accommodations. The client expressed ambivalence about the living arrangements and indicated that social isolation was beginning to be a major problem. The clinical nurse specialist encouraged the client to discuss feelings related to his living arrangements and suggested an increase in the present medication. Through the collaborative process with the client, the nurse, and the social worker in charge of the alternative living arrangement, the client agreed to continue weekly appointments at the mental health center.

Critical Thinking Issues

1. Discuss the positive symptoms associated with schizophrenia.

2. What cultural factors are known to affect the treatment of schizophrenia?

3. Discuss the psychosocial stressors that can precipitate the recurrence of schizophrenic symptoms.

4. Discuss the general goals of treatment for schizophrenia.

5. Discuss the importance of including the client and significant others in the treatment planning.

6. What effect will the collaboration process have on the client's response and progress?

Student Activities

The following statements describe behaviors commonly observed in persons diagnosed as having schizophrenia. Read each statement and categorize the behavior according to the following subtypes of schizophrenia: paranoid, disorganized, catatonic, undifferentiated, and residual.

1. Experiences unusual preoccupations
2. Hears "God's voice"; has no friends
3. Exhibits childlike behavior
4. Believes that the FBI is watching
5. Exhibits bizarre postures
6. Responds with "garbage walks voices talk."
7. Exhibits flat, blunt affect
8. Exhibits poor hygiene and self-care
9. Falsely accuses others
10. Expresses grandiose delusions
11. Exhibits inappropriate giggling
12. Maintains a motionless state

Answers

1. Residual
2 Undifferentiated
3. Disorganized
4. Paranoid
5. Catatonic
6. Catatonic
7. Residual
8. Undifferentiated
9. Paranoid
10. Paranoid
11. Disorganized
12. Catatonic

Characteristic Behaviors of Schizophrenia

- Positive Symptoms

  ▼ Hallucinations (distorted misperceptions of reality)

  ▼ Delusions (false beliefs)

  ▼ Formal Thought Disorders (disorganized speech, illogical thinking)

- Negative Symptoms

  ▼ Flat Affect

  ▼ Alogia

  ▼ Asociality

  ▼ Avolition

  ▼ Inattention

Developmental Phases of Schizophrenia

- Prodromal Phase (first phase)

  ▾ Social Withdrawal

  ▾ Work or School Impairment

  ▾ Lack of Motivation

  ▾ Poor Attention to Hygiene

  ▾ Strange Ideas

- Active Phase

  ▾ Delusions

  ▾ Hallucinations

  ▾ Disorganized Speech

  ▾ Catatonic Behavior

  ▾ Negative Symptoms

CHAPTER 19: Mood Disorders

Case Presentation

Brent is a 20-year-old college student. He was brought to the community mental health center after his roommates reported that he had not eaten or slept for the last week. He had been talking continuously, trying to convince them that he had found a scientific formula that would turn cigarette butts into gold. He knows that this will make him a multibillionaire, and he wants his roommates to share in his success and glory. Once his family arrives on the unit, his parents report that after graduating from high school, Brent was severely depressed and suicidal. An antidepressant was prescribed for him at that time. The family is very religious, and through his hospitalization and counseling with the pastor they survived his depressed period. During the initial assessment, the clinical nurse specialist performed a physical and mental status examination and determined that the client should be admitted for further observation and adjustment of his medication.

Critical Thinking Issues

1. Using the nursing process, develop a plan of care for Brent.

2. What is the priority nursing diagnosis for Brent?

3. What other nursing diagnosis would be appropriate?

4. How would the nurse use Brent's developmental stage in planning nursing care?

5. How would the nurse incorporate the family's strong religious beliefs into the plan of care?

6. What available community resources would be helpful for Brent?

Student Activities

Identify the following words or phrases that are all related to mood disorders. The letters marked with stars, once unscrambled, will reveal a priority nursing diagnosis for mood disorders.

Loss of pleasure

_ _ _ _ _ _ _ _
*   *

Rationale for use of anticonvulsant medications

_ _ _ _ _ _ _
    *

Chronic form of depression

_ _ _ _ _ _ _ _
  *

Increased sleep

_ _ _ _ _ _ _ _ _
   *   *

Depression rating scale

_ _ _ _
   *

Miscellaneous antidepressant medication

_ _ _ _ _ _ _ _ _
*   *

Treatment for seasonal affective disorder

_ _ _ _ _ _ _ _ _ _ _
        *

Seen in Bipolar II

_ _ _ _ _ _ _ _
   *

Speech pattern common in mania

_ _ _ _ _   _ _   _ _ _ _ _
  *   *

Alternative to lithium

_ _ _ _ _ _ _ _ _ _ _
*   *

Nursing diagnosis   _ _ _ _   _ _ _   _ _ _ _ _ _ _ _

Identify the following words or phrases that are all related to mood disorders. The letters marked with stars, once unscrambled, will reveal a priority nursing diagnosis for mood disorders.

Answers

Loss of pleasure
a n h e d o n i a
*   *

Rationale for use of anticonvulsant medications
k i n d l i n g
   *

Chronic form of depression
d y s t h y m i a
*

Increased sleep
h y p e r s o m n i a
   * *

Depression rating scale
B e c k
  *

Miscellaneous antidepressant medication
v e n l a f a x i n e
*   *

Treatment for seasonal affective disorder
p h o t o t h e r a p y
     *

Seen in Bipolar II
h y p o m a n i a
  *

Speech pattern common in mania
f l i g h t o f i d e a s
*   *

Alternative to lithium
c a r b a m a z e p i n e
* *

Nursing diagnosis   Risk for violence

109

Mood Disorders

Major Depression

- Definition

- Characteristic Behaviors

- Diagnostic Aids

- Culture, Age, and Gender Features

- Etiology

- Prognosis

- Assessment

- Planning Care

- Interventions for Hospitalized Clients

- Interventions for Clients in the Community

- Expected Outcomes

Bipolar Disorder

Characteristic Behaviors

- Diagnostic Aids

- Culture, Age, and Gender Features

- Etiology

- Prognosis

- Assessment

- Planning Care

- Interventions for Hospitalized Clients

- Interventions for Clients in the Community

- Client and Family Education

- Expected Outcomes

Differential Diagnosis

Common Nursing Diagnoses

CHAPTER 20: Anxiety Disorders

Case Presentation

Jamie Jenkins, a 19-year-old college student, went to the student health clinic complaining of shortness of breath, pounding heartbeat, and a marked feeling of apprehension. She stated, "I feel like I'm going to die!" These symptoms usually worsen during the times of examinations. Three weeks ago, her best friend dropped out of college. Her boyfriend broke up with her 6 weeks ago.

Critical Thinking Issues

1. What approach would be most therapeutic for the nurse to use during the initial interview with Jamie?

2. What questions must be asked initially?

3. Which factors may have precipitated the panic attacks?

4. What treatment approaches are indicated?

Student Activities

FIND-A-WORD PUZZLE

Hidden below are words related to Chapter 20. Circle each word that you find. The words may be found by searching across, up, down, forward, and backward. One word is selected as a sample.

AGORAPHOBIA
ANXIETY
BEHAVIOR
BIOFEEDBACK
BUSPAR
COGNITIVE
COMPULSIVE
DISORDER
ECT
GENERALIZED
IRRATIONAL
LOCUS OF CONTROL
MALADAPTIVE

MILD
OBSESSIVE
PANIC
PEPLAU
PHOBIA
POSTTRAUMATIC STRESS
PROGRESSIVE
RELAXATION
SEVERE
SOCIAL
SUPPORTIVE
VERBALIZE
THERAPY

```
P A N I C S O T X L N W A K C A B D E E F O I B C W
H N H A E L P O N S E G G S P G E D I E T A N D E D
O X C A L O Y N A H V P N I M O Z C A B N I L E O E
B I B M E A L A N X I O N A I R I I C C A N D E L A
I E V I T R O P P U S U G G E A L S T I V E L Y A A
A T E L E A D E N W S O K A L P A N D A S B E A R L
A Y E D O A G S E V E R E L L H B E L L T W O R E A
R S A I A U S A N T S K O O B O R A I A N B S X W E
E G G S A N D D A L B S C H K B E S A N D Y H O L R
D M E T I G H T A C O G N I T I V E P Y H E R A T R
R E E S T D N A X O W A L D L A E D P A R A D E S A
O T Y P E O V E R M N W O E E O R P O E N I A W S L
S A D Y K I O U A P G E I Z A L P U Y T S D E F A A
I L E A P E P L A U E B N I N E W R E A N Y A L L W
D O A N A V I L O L O U I L A I C O S S U A N N E S
A B C D E I F P O S T T R A U M A T I C S T R E S S
G H I J K T C E L I S T U R V W X Y A I B C O D E F
W B D F H P J L N V P R T E U W Y A B T C E I Q U I
Q W E R T A Y U R E I O P N A S D F G Y H J V K L Z
X C V B N D M N B V C X Z E L K J H G P F D A S A P
O B U S P A R I U Y T R E G W Q U E S A T I H O N S
A N S W E L O R T N O C F O S U C O L R R S E G O S
B E I R R A T I O N A L A T E O R O N E T I B M E F
O R P A R M T Y R O F N O E M O C W O H N E E D S A
P O E V I S S E R G O R P R E L A X A T I O N I P S
```

Puzzle Solution

```
P A N I C S O T X L N W A K C A B D E E F O I B C W
H N H A E L P O N S E G G S P G E D I E T A N D E D
O X C A L O Y N A H V P N I M O Z C A B N I L E O E
B I B M E A L A N X I O N A I R I I C C A N D E L A
I E V I T R O P P U S U G G E A L S T I V E L Y A A
A T E L E A D E N W S O K A L P A N D A S B E A R L
A Y E D O A G S E V E R E L L H B E L L T W O R E A
R S A I A U S A N T S K O O B O R A I A N B S X W E
E G G S A N D D A L B S C H K B E S A N D Y H O L R
D M E T I G H T A C O G N I T I V E P Y H E R A T R
R E E S T D N A X O W A L D L A E D P A R A D E S A
O T Y P E O V E R M N W O E E O R P O E N I A W S L
S A D Y K I O U A P G E I Z A L P U Y T S D E F A A
I L E A P E P L A U E B N I N E W R E A N Y A L L W
D O A N A V I L O L O U I L A I C O S S U A N N E S
A B C D E I F P O S T T R A U M A T I C S T R E S S
G H I J K T C E L I S T U R V W X Y A I B C O D E F
W B D F H P J L N V P R T E U W Y A B T C E I Q U I
Q W E R T A Y U R E I O P N A S D F G Y H J V K L Z
X C V B N D M N B V C X Z E L K J H G P F D A S A P
O B U S P A R I U Y T R E G W Q U E S A T I H O N S
A N S W E L O R T N O C F O S U C O L R R S E G O S
B E I R R A T I O N A L A T E O R O N E T I B M E F
O R P A R M T Y R O F N O E M O C W O H N E E D S A
P O E V I S S E R G O R P R E L A X A T I O N I P S
```

114

Anxiety Disorders

- Generalized Anxiety Disorder

- Panic Disorder with Agoraphobia

- Panic Disorder with Agoraphobia

- Agoraphobia

- Phobias

- Obsessive-Compulsive Disorder (OCD)

- Differential Diagnosis

  - Medical Disorders

  - Major Depression

  - Alcohol and Substance Abuse and Dependence

  - Personality Disorders

  - Posttraumatic Stress Disorder

CHAPTER 21: Somatoform Disorders

Case Presentation

A 25-year-old female college student sought medical attention for recurrent multiple somatic complaints. Her list of symptoms included gastrointestinal difficulties, painful menstruation, nausea, weakness, malaise, fatigue, headaches, back pain, and disturbed sleep. During the assessment, a complete history was taken of the current symptomatic complaints, associated symptoms, and behaviors. Information was also obtained about her childhood, family, education, and medical, and psychiatric treatment. The history revealed that she remembers a normal childhood and that she is close to her mother. Physical problems, which the client considered minor at that time, started during her last year of high school and continued to worsen to the present. Her mother took her to numerous physicians in an attempt to find solutions to her complaints. As a result, narcotics were prescribed and the client developed an addiction. Furthermore, exploratory laparotomies and multiple diagnostic procedures were performed, yet no organic cause was found. She expressed frustration that several doctors told her that she was a chronic complainer who didn't have anything wrong with her.

Critical Thinking Issues

1. What factors are associated with the development of somatization disorder?

2. Discuss the psychological meanings and messages in the symptoms exhibited by the client in the aforementioned scenario.

3. What is your response to clients who have no "real" physical disease?

4. What values are you aware of when intervening with clients who experience somatization disorder?

5. What are the most important nursing interventions for a client with somatization disorder?

Student Activities

In the following exercise, read each of the statements that are characteristic behaviors of somatoform disorders. Differentiate among somatization, undifferentiated somatoform disorder, conversion disorder, hypochondriasis, body dysmorphic disorder, and somatoform disorder not otherwise specified (NOS).

1. Complains of joint, abdominal, rectal, and chest pain.

2. Complains of fatigue, and loss of appetite that cannot be fully explained by a known general medical condition.

3. Manifests deafness after being told the marriage was over.

4. Focuses on "burning feet" and seeks help from several health-care providers even though no abnormal pathology was identified.

5. Focuses on facial wrinkles that are perceived as "ugly."

6. Exhibits signs and symptoms of pregnancy that include amenorrhea, breast enlargement, and secretions, but she is not pregnant.

7. Experiences severe migraine headaches during stressful events.

8. Experiences nausea, bloating, and diarrhea that cannot be fully explained by a known general medical condition.

9. Implements blood pressure testing several times per day to prevent other catastrophic medical conditions.

10. Describes a 6-month history of seeing many health-care providers and receiving numerous diagnostic tests.

11. Focuses excessively on facial freckles.

12. Exhibited a sudden paralysis of the arm. Medical work-ups ruled out organic conditions.

Answers

1. Somatization disorder
2. Undifferentiated somatoform disorder
3. Conversion disorder
4. Hypochondriasis
5. Body dysmorphic disorder
6. Somatoform disorder not otherwise specified (NOS)
7. Somatization disorder
8. Somatization disorder
9. Hypochondriasis
10. Hypochondriasis
11. Body dysmorphic disorder
12. Conversion disorder

Somatoform Disorders

- Somatization

- Undifferentiated Somatoform Disorder

- Conversion Disorder

- Pain Disorder

- Hypochondriasis

- Body Dysmorphic Disorder

CHAPTER 22: Post-Traumatic and Dissociative Disorders

Case Presentation

Ms. X, a 43-year-old woman and a mother of three children, was admitted to the psychiatric hospital with posttraumatic stress disorder (PTSD). She described her marriage as traumatic because of brutal sexual and physical treatment. She claimed that her ex-husband often held her at gun point during the sexual activity and threatened to kill her if she screamed or struggled. She had an 18-year history of symptoms of PTSD, which included nightmares, feelings of detachment, intrusive recollections of abuse, hypervigilance, insomnia, and irritability. She experienced significant disruptions in all aspects of her life. She had difficulty concentrating and experienced severe panic reactions. She denied alcohol abuse but acknowledged using anxiolytic agents excessively to ease the acute anxiety and panic attacks. Excessive drug use decreased her hypervigilance. Therapy was undertaken with mutually agreed upon goals. The first goal was to learn basic anxiety management techniques, which included relaxation, breathing control, and cognitive restructuring. The second goal was aimed at helping the client to identify and modify irrational-related beliefs that caused intense anxiety. The client agreed to keep a journal and discuss the contents during the therapy sessions.

Critical Thinking Issues

1. What predisposing factors are associated with the development of PTSD?

2. How does the experience of PTSD differ from the reaction to daily stress?

3. What are the most appropriate nursing interventions for the dissociating client?

4. Discuss the importance of homework assignments for the client with PTSD.

5. How does the behavior involved in PTSD differ from that of dissociative disorders?

Student Activity

1. During class, contrast and compare the various modalities relevant to PTSD.

2. Divide the class into groups of three to five students. Assign half of the groups to the task of formulating a list of major life issues that contribute to the development of PTSD. Assign the other half of the groups to the task of developing a teaching plan that will help a client identify potential triggers and manage intense anxiety. Ask students to share their results with the larger group.

Common Features of Posttraumatic Stress Disorder

- Aggressive Behavior

- Avoidance Behavior

- Constricted Affect

- Depression

- Detachment

- Guilty Rumination

- Hyperalertness

- Impulsiveness Insomnia

- Memory Impairment

- Nightmares

- Panic Attacks

- Phobic Responses

- Poor Concentration

- Repetitive Dreams

- Startle Reactions

CHAPTER 23: Sexual and Gender Identity Disorders

Case Presentation

Leslie, a 25-year-old man, discusses the sexual arousal and pleasure that he experiences while dressing as a woman. He also talks of how he purposefully brushes against others because of the thrill he receives. When asked about the onset of these behaviors, Leslie was unable to offer a specific time but stated that he had experienced these feelings as a teenager. He expresses a desire to rid himself of these feelings and wants to be "normal."

Critical Thinking Issues

1. Discuss how you would respond initially to Leslie's comments.

2. What would you tell Leslie about his feelings and behavior?

3. Identify one nursing diagnosis that is appropriate for Leslie.

4. Identify the interventions available to someone with Leslie's problems.

Student Activities

1. Define sexuality. Discuss your level of comfort with your own sexuality with your peers. Talk about your level of comfort with the sexuality of others.

2. Identify your role as a nurse when intervening with a person presenting with sexual dysfunction, gender identity problems, and paraphilias. Discuss your level of comfort with assessing and discussing details of a person's sex life. Are you judgmental?

3. Discuss what factors influence your beliefs and values regarding sexuality.

Sexual and Gender Identity Disorders

Normal Sexual Functioning in Men and Women

Sexual Dysfunction

- Characteristic Behaviors

- Culture, Age, and Gender Features

- Etiology

- Prognosis

- Interventions for Clients in the Community

Paraphilias

- Characteristic Behaviors

- Culture, Age, and Gender Features

- Etiology

- Prognosis

- Interventions for Clients in the Community

Client and Family Education

Expected Outcome

Common Nursing Diagnosis

CHAPTER 24: Eating Disorders

Case Presentation

Ms. T., a 23-year-old, referred herself to the eating disorder center at a prominent psychiatric hospital. During the assessment Ms. T. described fluctuations in her mood, but she was not aware that she had any significant health problems. She denied alcohol or drug abuse but acknowledged excessive laxative abuse. Initially, she was hesitant to talk about her eating problems. She stated, "I'm ashamed and embarrassed about my eating habits. I have a 3-year history of compulsive eating and binging of which my family is unaware. I have always had a weight control problem. I need treatment for binge eating and self-induced vomiting, which has happened every day for the past year." Ms T. added that when she experienced intense anxiety, she would binge and vomit more times than she could remember. The types of food that she consumed on a binge usually consisted of 3 quarts of ice cream, one large slice of chocolate cake, a bucket of buttered popcorn, eight chocolate candy bars, and two liters of regular soda. After eating approximately this amount of food, she would vomit. The nurse observed the following physical signs: calluses on the client's knuckles and a hoarseness when she talked. The client denied that amenorrhea was a problem. Ms. T. stated that she has become increasingly depressed, feels worthless, has low self-esteem, finds little pleasure in her work or family, and wonders whether life is worth living. She said that suicide is not an option, primarily because she feels that it would be unfair to her family. Food and weight concerns were used as a methods of coping with feelings of personal inadequacy.

Critical Thinking Issues

1. What are the goals of treatment for eating disorders?

2. Discuss the importance of involving the client in the treatment.

3. What are the life-threatening consequences of eating disorders?

4. How may the nurse assist the client with separation and individuation issues?

5. Discuss the usefulness of a contract with a bulimic client.

6. Discuss the similarities and differences between anorexia nervosa and bulimia nervosa in terms of clinical characteristics and nursing care.

Student Activities

1. Before class, ask students to write several questions related to the role(s) of the nurse in caring for a person with an eating disorder. During class period, have the students share the questions with the larger group. Provide time for discussion.

2. Generate a class discussion about factors that may contribute to the development of an eating disorder. Write the students' comments on an overhead transparency or on the chalkboard.
.
3. Below are words hidden in a puzzle. They may be read up, down, forward , backward, or diagonally, but always in a straight line. Some words may overlap, and some letters in the grid may be used more than once. Not all of the letters in the grid will be used. Circle the words that are listed.

FIND-A-WORD PUZZLE

ACIDOSIS	CONSTIPATION	INTENSE FEAR
ADOLESCENCE	DEHYDRATION	LANUGO
ALKALOSIS	DIURETICS	LAXATIVES
AMENORRHEA	DRY SKIN	VOMITING
ANEMIA	ENAMEL EROSION	WEIGHT GAIN
BINGING	HAIR LOSS	WEIGHT LOSS
BRITTLE HAIR	HYPOGLYCEMIA	WOMEN

```
H P B Y B V K O I S B V N L F
S Y F R S Z D G N S C O I A R
J I P U I B R U T O O M A X K
N Y S O A T S N E L N I G A S
D O B O G W T A N R S T T T Q
A S I W L L G L S I T I H I Y
M I N T O A Y N E A I N G V A
E S G F A M K C F H P G I E A
N O I S O R E L E M A N E S I
O D N R C W D N A M T I W K M
R I G N I K S Y R D I Z R B E
R C V Y G O B I H N O A V E N
H A A D O L E S C E N C E Z A
E T S C I T E R U I D A N G T
A T I S S O L T H G I E W J T
```

Puzzle Solution

```
H P B Y B V K O I S B V N L F
S Y F R S Z D G N S C O I A R
J I P U I B R U T O O M A X K
N Y S O A T S N E L N I G A S
D O B O G W T A N R S T T T Q
A S I W L L G L S I T I H I Y
M I N T O A Y N E A I N G V A
E S G F A M K C F H P G I E A
N O I S O R E L E M A N E S I
O D N R C W D N A M T I W K M
R I G N I K S Y R D I Z R B E
R C V Y G O B I H N O A V E N
H A A D O L E S C E N C E Z A
E T S C I T E R U I D A N G T
A T I S S O L T H G I E W J T
```

Types of Eating Disorders

- Anorexia Nervosa

- Bulimia Nervosa

- Binge Eating Disorder

CHAPTER 25: Sleep Disorders

Case Presentation

A 55-year-old married white woman presented with chief complaints of sleep disturbance at night and fatigue during the day. Because of her sleep-wake cycle, she was referred to the sleep disorder clinic. She stated that her insomnia had worsened over the past 2 years. She stated that she was alert in the late evening; had difficulty falling asleep; and awoke frequently during the night.She had no problem awakening in the morning. It was difficult for her to fall asleep, because she found herself ruminating about the years of sexual abuse that occurred during her childhood and also about her husband's loud snoring. She described having vivid, recurrent, distressing dreams at night. These dreams were related to her years as a victim of sexual abuse, which included fondling and penetration, and the dreams were accompanied by a profound sense of helplessness. When awakening in the morning, the client described low energy, fatigue, and sleepiness. The client recorded her sleep pattern on the sleep evaluation log, and antidepressants were prescribed to her as a result of the psychological and psychiatric assessment, which suggested a depressive disorder. She experienced complete relief of her sleep schedule.

Critical Thinking Issues

1. What is the personal impact of an untreated sleep disorder?

2. What are the goals for a client experiencing a sleep disorder?

3. What are the most appropriate nursing interventions for a client with insomnia?

4. What interventions promote a healthy sleep-wake pattern?

Student Activities

Match the statements in column I with the appropriate description in column II.

Column I

A. Central sleep apnea

B. Circadian rhythmicity

C. Dyssomnia

D. Hypersomnia

E. Narcolepsy

F. Obstructive sleep apnea

G. Parasomnia

H. Phase-advanced sleep pattern

I. Rapid eye movement (REM) sleep

J. Sleep diary

K. Sleep hygiene

L. Sleep-wake cycle

M. Circadian rhythm sleep disorder

Column II

___Characterized by excess sleep, with long periods during the night

___Plays a major role in sleep onset

___Actual eye movements, atonia, and dreaming

___Early to bed at 7:00 PM and waking early about 3:00 AM

___Disorder characterized by either insomnia or hypersomnia

___Abnormal behaviors linked to sleep or sleep-wake transitions

___Healthy sleep-wake patterns

___Frequent nighttime arousals and daytime sleepiness

___Follows a 24-hour or circadian pattern

___ Short periods of irresistible sleepiness daily, lasting for 3 months

___Difficulty in initiating or maintaining sleep

___Documenting the exact sleep-wake pattern and disruptions

___The upper airway becomes partially or completely obstructed

Answers

Column I	**Column II**

Column I

A. Central sleep apnea

B. Circadian rhythmicity

C. Dyssomnia

D. Hypersomnia

E. Narcolepsy

F. Obstructive sleep apnea

G. Parasomnia

H. Phase-advanced sleep pattern

I. Rapid eye movement sleep (REM)

J. Sleep diary

K. Sleep hygiene

L. Sleep-wake cycle

M. Circadian rhythm sleep disorder

Column II

D Characterized by excess sleep, with long periods during the night

B Plays a major role in sleep onset

I Actual eye movements, atonia, and dreaming

H Early to bed at 7:00 PM and waking early about 3:00 AM

M Disorder characterized by either insomnia or hypersomnia

G Abnormal behaviors linked to sleep, or sleep-wake transitions

K Behaviors that promote healthy sleep-wake patterns

A Frequent nighttime arousals and daytime sleepiness

L Follows a 24-hour or circadian pattern

E Short periods of irresistible sleepiness daily, lasting for 3 months

C Difficulty in initiating or maintaining sleep

J Documenting the exact sleep-wake pattern and disruptions

F The upper airway becomes partially or completely obstructed

Sleep Disorders

- Primary Insomnia

- Primary Hypersomnia

- Breathing-Related Sleep Disorders

- Narcolepsy

- Circadian Rhythm Sleep Disorder

- Dyssomnia Not Otherwise Specified (NOS)

- Parasomnias

- Differential Diagnosis

  - Sleep Disorder Due to a General Medical Condition

  - Substance-Induced Sleep Disorder

  - Mood Disorders

  - Anxiety Disorders

CHAPTER 26: Adjustment Disorders

Case Presentation

Jennie, a 45-year-old divorced woman, presented to the community mental health clinic with depression. She described symptoms of long-standing depression that included a negative view of self, her present situation, and the future. She described her level of emotions as mild to moderate feelings of hopelessness and sadness. She recently experienced several stressors within a short period of time and was finding it difficult to maintain a balanced view of self and the future. She stated that her childhood was chaotic and unhappy. She had feelings of distress and frustration, and she remembers crying a lot. Her sleep pattern was a problem because of excessive worrying and negative thinking about lack of nurturance and consistency in her life. She described her relationship with her mother as poor owing to communication problems and lack of affection, but she got along with her siblings and felt close to them. Because of an alcoholic father, a disruptive environment was always present. She never developed friendships at school, because she felt that she never fit in. She stated that each new situation brought back old feelings and behaviors. On the mental status examination, she presented as a large woman of average weight and stated age. Her personal hygiene was neat and well groomed. She responded pleasantly and cooperatively during the intake process and did not seem particularly anxious. Her speech was clear and coherent and had a normal rhythm and tone. Her thought content was focused on the overall depression, and her problem-solving abilities were marginally functional. Throughout the interview she displayed a full range of affect. She was oriented to time, place, person, and situation. Her recent and remote memories were intact. She displayed no history of psychosis.

Critical Thinking Issues

1. What are the factors that precipitate emotional problems for persons experiencing adjustment disorder?

2. Discuss the importance of a collaborative relationship.

3. Develop two nursing diagnoses related to the above scenario.

4. Discuss the most appropriate nursing interventions that will help solve the client's problems.

5. Identify the projected, realistic client outcomes, and individualize them to the client's situation.

Student Activities

1. Before class, instruct each student to research articles related to coping strategies or psychological adaptation. Divide the class into groups of four or five students and, within each group, have the students compare and contrast the findings of each study. Ask the groups to share the information with the entire class group.

2. Divide the class into groups of 8 to 10 students, and ask each group to form a circle. Have each student develop a scenario about a stressful event that took place during his or her lifetime, and write it on an 8½ by 11" sheet of paper. After completion of this task, instruct the students in each group to fold the paper in half and place it on the floor in the middle of the circle. Then ask each student to randomly select one of the folded papers and, after reading the scenario, have him or her respond by writing the necessary coping strategies that may help the person adjust to the stress. Place the folded papers back on the floor in the middle of the circle. Instruct students to randomly select one piece of paper and, one at a time, read the scenario and the coping strategies. Allow time for discussion between each participant.

3. If available, provide each student with The Social Readjustment Rating Scale by Holmes and Rahe. Provide class time for the students to evaluate their life events. Allow time for discussion.

Adjustment Disorders

- Differential Diagnosis

  ▾ Mood Disorders

  ▾ Posttraumatic Stress Disorders

  ▾ Acute Stress Disorder

  ▾ Bereavement

CHAPTER 27: Personality Disorders

Case Presentation

L., a 32-year-old white woman who is the mother of a 6-year-old daughter, was recently separated from her husband with whom she had a series of violent arguments. She was admitted to the emergency room because of self-inflicted razor cuts to her wrists, which she claimed made her feel alive by feeling pain. She was referred to the psychiatric unit of the hospital because she stated that she intended to commit suicide. On admission, the clinical nurse specialist (CNS) attempted to interview L. Initially, the client was uncooperative and felt abandoned by society and especially by her husband, because he had full custody of her daughter and was living with another woman who was taking care of her child. She was angry about the arrangement and claimed that she did not really love her husband, but that she needed him to take care of her. She is convinced that one day he will take her back; however, in the interim, she will have to return to the care of father to whom she feels very close. She admitted to the excessive use of anxiolytics and alcohol to control her anxiety and numb the emotional pain. Her presenting complaints consisted of angry outbursts, feelings of emptiness, rejection, loneliness, and depression. She states that she has difficulty getting along with people and experiences rapid mood swings involving depression, anger, and anxiety. She has periods when she feels good about herself and practices self-care. At other times, she finds it impossible to get out of bed and take care of anything. She lacks a sense of identity and doesn't really know who she is from one minute to the next. During hospitalization the treatment focused on reduction of the imminent threat to L.'s life and on helping her to develop more effective coping strategies. L. was assigned to a primary nurse who set limits on her behavior and agreed to help her manage her patterns of emotional instability. Due to limited psychiatric hospitalization, L. was discharged in 5 days with a diagnosis of borderline personality disorder. The client was referred for individual therapy with a CNS.

Critical Thinking Issues

1. What are realistic short-term goals for a hospitalized client with borderline personality disorder?

2. How does a personality disorder affect a person's relationships and overall well-being?

3. What are the most appropriate nursing interventions for the hospitalized client with a personality disorder?

4. What strategies encourage an individual with a personality disorder to seek psychiatric treatment?

5. Design a plan of care that includes the nursing diagnosis, interventions, and outcomes for a client diagnosed as having a borderline personality disorder.

Student Activities

Match the personality characteristics in column I with the appropriate disorder in column II.

Column I

A. Suspicious and mistrustful

B. As a child, displayed conduct problems such as assault and cruelty to animals

C. Unstable and intense interpersonal relationships

D. Lacks social and close relationships and has difficulty relating to others

E. Feelings are often excessive, shallow, changeable, and short-lived

F. Manipulative and demanding

G. Has difficulty forming intimate relationships

H. Good and bad views of the world

I. Long-standing pattern of lack of concern for and violation of the rights of others

J. Always seeking attention

K. Suspicious, lacks friends, and displays inappropriate affect

L. Shifts from admiring, liking, and even loving the other person to devaluing and hating him or her

M. Unable to form secure relationships and frantically avoids real or imagined loss

Column II

___Schizoid Personality Disorder

___Paranoid Personality Disorder

___Paranoid Personality Disorder

___Antisocial Personality Disorder

___Schizotypical Personality Disorder

___Histrionic Personality Disorder

___Borderline Personality Disorder

___Narcissistic Personality Disorder

___Avoidant Personality Disorder

___Borderline Personality Disorder

___Antisocial Personality Disorder

___Dependent Personality Disorder

___Obsessive-Compulsive Personality Disorder

N. Wants desperately to be noticed and loved

O. Often does not feel remorseful over the harm or pain that he or she causes

P. Displays behaviors that seem like a milder, nonpsychotic state of schizophrenia

Q. Extremely shy, self-conscious, and awkward

R. Extreme sense of arrogance, entitlement, and self-importance.

S. Shows an overreliance on others for support, reassurance, and love

T. Confronted with extreme anxiety and fear in social and intimate relationships

U. Extreme rigidity and control

V. Unable to make decisions and expects friends and families to make them

W. Driven by "self-love" and takes advantage of others

X. Overly organized, and pays extreme attention to detail.

Z. Has tremendous difficulty in work situations and intimate relationships.

___Obsessive-Compulsive Personality Disorder

___Dependent Personality Disorder

___Avoidant Personality Disorder

___Borderline Personality Disorder

___Schizotypal Personality Disorder

___Histrionic Personality Disorder

___Antisocial Personality Disorder

___Narcissistic Personality Disorder

___Borderline Personality Disorder

___Histrionic Personality Disorder

___Borderline Personality Disorder

___Obsessive-Compulsive Personality Disorder

Answers

Column I	Column II
A. Suspicious and mistrustful	D Schizoid Personality Disorder
B. As a child, displayed conduct problems, such as assaults and cruelty to animals	A Paranoid Personality Disorder
C. Unstable and intense interpersonal relationships	G Paranoid Personality Disorder
D. Lacks social and close relationships and has difficulty relating to others	I Antisocial Personality Disorder
E. Feelings are often excessive, shallow, changeable, and short-lived	K Schizotypical Personality Disorder
F. Manipulative and demanding	J Histrionic Personality Disorder
G. Has difficulty forming intimate relationships	C Borderline Personality Disorder
H. Good and bad views of the world	W Narcissistic Personality Disorder
I. Long-standing pattern of lack of concern for and violation of the rights of others	Q Avoidant Personality Disorder
J. Always seeking attention	F Borderline Personality Disorder
K. Suspicious, lacks friends, and displays inappropriate affect	O Antisocial Personality Disorder
L. Shifts from admiring, liking, and even loving the other person to devaluing and hating him or her	S Dependent Personality Disorder
M. Unable to form secure relationships, and frantically avoids real or imagined loss	Z Obsessive-Compulsive Personality Disorder

N. Wants desperately to be noticed and loved

O. Often does not feel remorseful over the harm or pain that he or she causes

P. Displays behaviors that seem like a milder, nonpsychotic state of schizophrenia

Q. Extremely shy, self-conscious, and awkward

R. Extreme sense of arrogance, entitlement, and self-importance

S. Shows an overreliance on others for support, reassurance, and love

T. Confronted with extreme anxiety and fear in social and intimate relationships

U. Extreme rigidity and control

V. Unable to make decisions and expects friends and families to make them

W. Driven by "self-love" and takes advantage of others

X. Overly organized and pays extreme attention to detail

Z. Has tremendous difficulty in work situations and intimate relationships

X_Obsessive-Compulsive Personality Disorder

V_Dependent Personality Disorder

T_Avoidant Personality Disorder

M_Borderline Personality Disorder

P_Schizotypal Personality Disorder

N_Histrionic Personality Disorder

B_Antisocial Personality Disorder

R_Narcissistic Personality Disorder

L_Borderline Personality Disorder

E_Histrionic Personality Disorder

H_Borderline Personality Disorder

U_Obsessive-Compulsive Personality Disorder

Personality Disorders

Cluster A Personality Disorders

- Paranoid

- Schizotypal

- Schizoid

Cluster B Personality Disorders

- Antisocial

- Borderline

- Histrionic

- Narcissistic

Cluster C Personality Disorders

- Avoidant Personality Disorder

- Dependent Personality Disorder

- Obsessive-Compulsive Personality Disorder

CHAPTER 28: Attention-Deficit Hyperactivity Disorder

Case Presentation

James, a 13-year-old boy who was living in a group home, was admitted to the adolescent unit for evaluation because of an increase in hyperactive, oppositional, and disruptive behavior. According to his group home parents, James had excessive energy, difficulty with task completion, and repeated physical fights with other group home members. He was irritable, intrusive, and easily distracted, and he destroyed property when he was angry. James exhibited similar behavior during his school day program. The teacher's report cited a major problem with attitude and severe behavioral problems that impaired his school performance. The report indicated that he was uncooperative, disruptive, and impulsive and that he did not listen to instructions. He had difficulty waiting his turn; he was unable to sit still for any length of time; and his school performance was impaired. During the assessment, James, who appeared his stated age, presented as a well-oriented, bright 13-year-old. Initially, he refused to talk with the clinical nurse specialist. Once he felt comfortable, he cooperated and answered all questions willingly and spontaneously. He was able to remain seated throughout the interview and appeared attentive during the discussion. At times, he fidgeted with his hands and squirmed in his seat, reporting that he was "nervous." He spoke clearly and coherently using normal rate and tone. His mood was slightly anxious, with some sadness noted when discussing his problems. He admitted feeling sad at times because his parents had abandoned him, and he did not know where they were living or if they were even alive. He talked about his interactions with peers at the group home and at school, which were frequently antagonistic and resulted in verbal and physical fights. His intellect and memory were adequate, and his knowledge of general information seemed average. He did not exhibit concern regarding his poor school performance. James was diagnosed as having attention-deficit hyperactivity disorder (ADHD). The multidisciplinary team plan was designed and implemented. The planned approach was to actively involve the group home parents, implement behavioral techniques to decrease maladaptive behaviors, explore strengths, increase his sense of self-esteem, and teach adaptive and effective coping strategies.

Critical Thinking Issues

1. What assumptions can you conclude from this case presentation?

2. Discuss the importance of reframing behavior.

3. How can the nurse assist the teacher in providing structure within the school environment?

4. How can the nurse assist the group home parent with reinforcement of positive behaviors?

5. Design a plan of care including the nursing diagnosis, interventions, and outcomes.

Student Activities

1. Ask students in the class who have encountered or currently know a child, adolescent, or adult diagnosed as having ADHD to share their observations about the individual's behavior. Generate a discussion about the characteristics, and compare the students' observations with the diagnostic criteria listed in this chapter.
2. Divide the class into groups of six to eight students, and provide 4 x 6" index cards to each student. Assign two groups to write DSM-IV criteria for ADHD. On a one-group-per-task basis, assign the remaining groups the following writing tasks.

    a. Describe the clinical presentation of ADHD symptoms in children.
    b. Describe the clinical presentation of ADHD in adolescents.
    c. Describe the clinical presentation of ADHD in the adult.
    d. List the impact of ADHD on the social functioning of the child.
    e. List the impact of ADHD on the social functioning of the adolescent.
    f. List the impact of ADHD on the social functioning of the adult.

The components of each task may be divided among the students in each group. Generate a discussion about the information acquired by the students, and include culture, age, and gender issues. Discuss the roles of the nurse when planning care for the client with ADHD.

Attention-Deficit Hyperactivity Disorder

Characteristic Behaviors

Children

- Inattention

- Hyperactivity

- Impulsivity

Adolescents

- May deny or make excuses

Adults

- Emphasize difficulty with increased expectations and responsibilities

CHAPTER 29: Prolonged Mental Illness: Clients and Their Families in the Community

Case Presentation

Louise is a 68-year-old woman with a 35-year history of bipolar disorder. After a recent hospitalization, Louise is being seen by a psychiatric home care nurse. Louise lives in a small apartment, which is cluttered and dirty. There are numerous empty containers of snack foods in the kitchen and bedroom. Louise does not drive but lives close to a city bus route and has a convenience store at the corner of her block. Her daughter lives in the same city and makes telephone contact with her once or twice a week. Louise's landlord assists her with obtaining medication and groceries. She has a history of not following her prescribed schedule of medications, which include lithium. Her behavior is illustrated by the following statements. "I don't know what all the fuss is about. I'm perfectly able to take care of myself. Who said I don't take my medicine? Look, I have this box that holds all my pills. My landlord helps me fill it every week. You say it's Wednesday? I don't know why Tuesday is still filled with medicine. Oh well, look around if you want to but I don't need anything. I have bread and luncheon meat to make sandwiches and plenty of snacks. Would you care for a cookie? My daughter called today. She said that she might be able to stop by later with some milk. She's got her hands full, you know---with that husband of hers. You're welcome to come back if you want; just remember that I don't get up until about noon. I usually fall asleep watching the late, late movie."

Critical Thinking Issues

1. What assumptions might be made about Louise after reading her story?

2. What assumptions might be made related to her daughter?

3. What assumptions might be made related to her landlord?

4. What are the characteristics of prolonged mental illness that are exhibited by Louise?

5. How can Louise be assisted in gaining insight regarding her present situation?

6. What defense mechanism is she presently using?

7. Discuss other health risk factors that Louise may be experiencing.

8. What questions might be asked of Louise's daughter and landlord to obtain relevant information about family and support systems?

9. Identify at lease two community resources that might assist Louise in coping with prolonged mental illness.

10. Describe a model of treatment and rehabilitation that would be appropriate for Louise and her daughter.

Student Activities

1. Assign students to investigate a community resource that is available to a client with prolonged mental illness, and assess its effectiveness in meeting the needs of the client.

2. Develop a plan of care for Louise utilizing a continuous treatment plan of approach.

3. Interview a client with prolonged mental illness and ask about his or her experience of stigma.

4. Present the students with an ethical dilemma related to managed costs and rationed care. Instruct the students to research the topic prior to class and be prepared to discuss society's unwillingness to underwrite psychiatric costs for mental illness. Also include in the discussion fewer professionals and more untrained and unlicensed staff who are in charge of client care.

Prolonged Mental Illness: Clients and Their Families in the Community

- Characteristics of Prolonged Mental Illness

- Impact of Prolonged Mental Illness

- Models of Treatment and Rehabilitation

  ▾ Case Management

  ▾ Continuous Treatment Teams

  ▾ Residential Care

  ▾ Psychosocial Rehabilitation Programs

CHAPTER 30: The Faces of Homelessness

Case Presentation

Mr. B. was a 43-year-old Vietnam veteran who presented at the homeless clinic with a long-standing history of substance abuse. He was seeking help for physical problems caused by the rigors of street living and after years of substance abuse and physical problems. During the initial evaluation, he reported that he continued to use marijuana, alcohol, and cocaine. Cocaine was his drug of choice, and he would do anything to obtain it. B. presented as dirty, unshaven, and malodorous, and his clothes were in a state of disrepair. He appeared older than his stated age. His posture was slumped; he maintained eye contact; and he was alert and oriented in all four spheres. He reported feeling anxious, hopeless, and worthless. He admitted that he had no personal goals. He was not looking forward to a successful future; instead, he was just trying to survive on a daily basis. B. stated that he was from a middle-class family and that he was the fourth of seven children. He experienced much criticism in his youth and described his father as a strict disciplinarian. B. left home at the age of 18. He enlisted in the military and served for 4 years in Vietnam. During this time in Vietnam, he became addicted to numerous substances. Upon returning to the United States and to his family, he was addicted to cocaine and was unable to maintain a job. While attempting to support his addiction to cocaine, he stole from his immediate family and then from small businesses until he was caught and sent to jail. When he was released from jail, he lived on the street for 2 years until his physical health started to deteriorate. The physical assessment indicated hypertension, peripheral vascular disease, and diabetes type I. On examination of the legs and feet, the nurse found multiple ulcers that were draining copious, purulent, foul-smelling discharge. The client reported that the pain was excruciating and made it difficult for him to walk. Nursing care was initiated to promote ulcer healing and provide shelter until a more permanent housing arrangement could be made.

Critical Thinking Issues

1. Using the nursing assessment, identify specific areas for further investigation.

2. How does living on the street affect people?

3. Discuss how B. is coping with life events.

4. What are the most appropriate nursing interventions for B.'s substance abuse?

5. Discuss prioritizing interventions to deal with the client's physical problems.

6. How do health-care professionals help the homeless client to improve conditions of daily living?

7. Identify additional resources or service providers that would assist in Mr. B.'s mental health.

Student Activities

Word-Find Puzzle

Below are words hidden in the puzzle. They may be read up, down, forward, backward, or diagonally, but always in a straight line. Some words may overlap, and some letters in the grid may be used more than once. Not all letters in the grid will be used. Circle each word as you locate it.

ABUSE	GENTRIFICATION	PROFESSIONAL
ADOLESCENTS	HEALTH-CARE DELIVERY	RAPE
ADVOCACY	HOMELESS	RECENT HOMELESS
ALCOHOL	MALE	REST
BEHAVIORS	MALIGNANT	SHELTERS
BENIGN	MALNOURISHED	SOCIAL DISTRESS
CHILDREN	MARGINAL	SOCIOECONOMIC
CLINIC	MENTALLY ILL	SOUP KITCHEN
COGNITIVE	MISSIONS	STEALING
CONDITIONS	MOOD	STRATEGIES
COPING SKILLS	NURSE	STREETS
DEINDUSTRIALIZATION	NUTRITION	SUBGROUPS
EMERGENCIES	OLD	SUBSTANCE ABUSE
FEET	ORIENTED	ULCERS
FLOPHOUSES	POLITICAL	VASCULAR DISEASE
		WEATHER

```
P Y R E V I L E D E R A C H Y L A E H L
X S M P U E S A E S I D R A L U C S A V
P H A R S C O P I N G S K I L L S O D P
S E L O E I B E N I G N S F E E T C O E
E L I F S C G U D M U N U G R W R I L M
I T G E U U E N E R E E B T G E S O E E
G E N S O X N N S C P N S A H J R E S R
E R A S H B T E T A O I T T H Y E C C G
T S N I P E R R R H D G A A C E C O E E
A E T O O H I D I L O E N A L N L N N N
R Y L N L A F L A T W M C I I L U O T C
T L A A F V I I L R K O E B T O Y M S I
S A N L M I C H I Z V O A L O I G I O E
T C I C M O A C Z D M D B H E H V C L S
E I G O S R T M A L N O U R I S H E D L
A T R H F S I G T V Q I S N O I S S I M
L I A O F I O R I E N T E D C I N I L C
I L M L E J N C O N D I T I O N S S Q R
N O I T I R T U N E H C T I K P U O S G
G P S U B G R O U P S T E E R T S E R E
```

Answers

148

```
P Y R E V I L E D E R A C H Y L A E H L
X S M P U E S A E S I D R A L U C S A V
P H A R S C O P I N G S K I L L S O D P
S E L O E I B E N I G N S F E E T C O E
E L I F S C G U D M U N U G R W R I L M
I T G E U U E N E R E E B T G E S O E E
G E N S O X N N S C P N S A H J R E S R
E R A S H B T E T A O I T T H Y E C C G
T S N I P E R R R H D G A A C E C O E E
A E T O O H I D I L O E N A L N L N N N
R Y L N L A F L A T W M C I I L U O T C
T L A A F V I I L R K O E B T O Y M S I
S A N L M I C H I Z V O A L O I G I O E
T C I C M O A C Z D M D B H E H V C L S
E I G O S R T M A L N O U R I S H E D L
A T R H F S I G T V Q I S N O I S S I M
L I A O F I O R I E N T E D C I N I L C
I L M L E J N C O N D I T I O N S S Q R
N O I T I R T U N E H C T I K P U O S G
G P S U B G R O U P S T E E R T S E R E
```

1. Visit a homeless shelter and interview a homeless person. Develop a care plan using the nursing process.

2. Invite a nurse or legal expert to share his or her knowledge about the homeless population.

3. Generate a discussion about society's approach to the homeless population, and include society's attitudes and values and economic issues in the discussion.

Psychiatric–Mental Health Nursing and the Homeless

- Historical Background

- Theoretical Basis for Nursing Practice

- Psychiatric–Mental Health Nursing Intervention Strategies

- Advocacy Role for the Homeless

CHAPTER 31: Victims of Sexual Abuse

Case Presentation

Seven-year-old May was brought to the emergency room by her mother and her mother's live-in boyfriend with complaints of a reddened and painful vaginal area. On examination, the vaginal area was swollen and had small lacerations. May's mother's boyfriend volunteered that the injury was caused when May fell off her bicycle. Each time that a question was directed to May or to the mother, the boyfriend would respond. The nurse also noted that the child was quiet and withdrawn and failed to make eye contact with the mother.

Critical Thinking Issues

1. Identify the behaviors in this situation that are suggestive of abuse.

2. Why is it important for the nurse to ask direct questions regarding the possibility of abuse?

3. What could the nurse do to elicit direct responses from the child and the mother?

4. What must you do if you suspect abuse?

5. Identify the priority intervention to be used with May.

6. Identify future problems that abused children are at greater risk of developing.

7. Identify at least two nursing diagnoses that are appropriate for May's situation.

Student Activities

1. Identify two resources in your community that are available to victims of sexual abuse. What services are provided by these agencies? Who pays for these services? How should referrals be made to these agencies?

2. Call the child protection agency in your state and inquire about procedures for handling a report of potential sexual abuse.

3. Contact a minimum of three hospitals in your state and find out what policy exists for reporting suspected cases of sexual abuse.

4. Find out about the law in your state regarding your role in reporting sexual abuse.

Victims of Abuse

Types of Abuse

- Physical Abuse

- Sexual Abuse

- Economic Abuse

Components of Abuse

- Perpetrator

- Violence in the Home

- Violence in the Environment

- Survivor

Trauma Responses

Assessment of Abuse

- Indicators

- Abuse-Related Symptoms

Key Principles of Treatment

- Maintain Safety

- Empower the Individual

- Report by Mandated Law

- Minimize Intrusiveness

- Keep Secrets

- Identify Symptom Clusters

- Know Your Level of Expertise

- Do Not Pathologize

- Do Not Reinforce Perceptions of Shame or Vulnerability

- Be Aware of Possible Cognitive Distortions

Treatment of Abuse Victims

- Individual Psychotherapy

- Group Psychotherapy

- Family, Couples, and Sex Therapy

- Pharmacologic Treatment

- Potential Countertransference

CHAPTER 32: Persons Living with HIV Disease/AIDS

Case Presentation

Mr. B., a 28-year-old executive assistant, attended night school to complete his undergraduate business administration degree. He described his troubles during his adolescent years. He was teased by his peers for being effeminate and for having a small body. His sexual relationships were exclusively homosexual and had all been unsatisfactory. After leaving home, he dated several girls and lived with a girlfriend for approximately 1 year. He reported that although he enjoyed his girlfriend's company and adopted the role of keeping her happy, the relationship had not been particularly fulfilling sexually or emotionally. The client began to realize that he wanted to be more attractive to other men and stated that he felt significantly more emotional and sexually connected with men than women. He started to date a male classmate, and shortly thereafter they moved in together. The relationship proved to be congenial and supportive, and both persons were satisfied with their sexual and emotional relationship. Within a year of their living arrangement, the client described fluctuations in mood and developed extreme lethargy, insomnia, lack of appetite, depression, and dysthymia. The client sought medical help to deal with his physical problems. Following a psychosocial history and a review of Mr. B.'s medical history, he was tested for the human immunodeficiency virus (HIV). The test report was positive for HIV. The client experienced shock and denial that he had contracted this life-threatening illness. His fear, anger, depression, and isolation increased during the next few months. Mr. B. and his partner were fearful that they would be ostracized by friends and workmates. They both expressed feelings of entrapment and mourned the losses that they were about to encounter. Mr. B. isolated himself from social activities in fear of rejection. While Mr. B. underwent treatment for HIV and therapy for his psychological problems, he relinquished his night school activity but continued to work as an executive assistant. He experienced severe physical problems, lethargy, and diminished thought processes. When his energy decreased, he reduced his work day hours. The psychiatric clinical nurse specialist provided supportive therapy sessions to help Mr. B. to deal with issues regarding his state of health, losses, self-esteem, isolation, and anger.

Critical Thinking Issues

1. What is the role of the psychiatric nurse in taking care of Mr. B.?

2. What nursing interventions are most likely to be provided for Mr. B.?

3. What assumptions can you make about Mr. B.'s psychosocial history?

4. What assumptions can you make about Mr. B.'s supportive therapy?

Student Activities

1. Tell the students that an epidemic of the acquired immunodeficiency syndrome (AIDS) has occurred in the city of Charm, and they are all members of the group diagnosed with the disease. Instruct them to draw a straight horizontal line on an 8½ x 11" sheet of paper. Place a dot at each end of the line. Over the dot on the left side of the line, place the date of the activity. Over the dot on the right side of the line, place the year that you expect to die of the disease. After allowing the students time to reflect, ask the students to share their feelings. Encourage a discussion about coping with present daily life and regarding hope for the future.

2. Generate a discussion related to the students' beliefs about HIV and AIDS.

3. Interview a client with AIDS. Collect the data, and then develop a nursing care plan that includes available community support systems.

4. Assign a group of students to investigate and evaluate community resources available for persons with AIDS.

Persons Living with HIV and AIDS

Mode of Transmission

Epidemiology

Clinical Manifestation and the Spectrum of HIV Diseases

- Early Stage

- Middle Stage

- Late Stage

Neuropsychological Complications

Other Psychiatric Disorders

Patient Care

- Assessment

- Nursing Diagnosis

- Planning and Therapeutics

- Hope for the Future: Protease Inhibitors

Vulnerable Populations

- The Severely and Persistently Mentally Ill

- Women

- Substance Abusers

CHAPTER 33: Persons in Correctional Facilities

Case Presentation

Orgamy is a 30-year-old woman committed to a state maximum security correctional institution for substance abuse, cocaine trafficking, assault, and second-degree murder. Her history revealed that she grew up in a single-parent home and that she was one of three children. Her mother was poorly educated and found job placement difficult. Her mother moved the impoverished family from one town to another in her search for employment. Orgamy left home to make a life of her own when she was 14 years of age. During this period, she failed to develop relationships and exploited others for personal gain. A mental status examination was completed in which she exhibited a low tolerance for frustration and during which she was brusque, belligerent, exploitative, and manipulative. She often intimidated the other inmates with her argumentative, malicious, cold, and callous behavior. During the early part of her incarceration, she attempted to break the rules and used inappropriate language when addressing the health-care team, members of the correctional institution, and fellow inmates. Her intimidating behavior toward her fellow inmates created friction, and an assault ensued. She incurred a fracture of the right hand, multiple rib fractures, lacerations, and abrasions. She received emergency care and was hospitalized in the prison in-patient unit. It was later learned that she had a child whom she abused physically, and she allowed the child to be sexually abused by her male acquaintances. Orgamy was referred to a psychiatric clinical nurse specialist for further evaluation. She was diagnosed as having antisocial personality disorder, and she was admitted to the psychiatric unit in the prison. A multifaceted treatment approach, including individual and group therapy, was used. During the group sessions, Orgamy always saw herself as a victim and refused to accept responsibility for the consequences of her behavior. Individual sessions were unproductive.

Critical Thinking Issues

1. What additional data would you obtain from Orgamy?

2. List the significant assessment findings.

3. What nursing interventions would be most effective to help Orgamy?

4. Does an inmate feel dehumanized? Discuss Orgamy's ability to feel dehumanized.

5. How would you judge Orgamy for her crimes?

7. How would you approach an inmate who harbors debilitating hate and distrust?

Student Activities

1. Visualize yourself as part of the mental health disciplinary team in a maximum security correctional institution. Describe your feelings.

2. How would you plan mental health care for a long-term inmate?

3. Describe how you would implement your plan of care while security personnel try to maintain a safe environment.

4. In small groups of six or eight students, discuss the positive and negative aspects of an adequate and safe mental health delivery system in a correctional institution.

5. Each culture has its own values. Discuss how values are different or the same with each culture.

6. Identify health beliefs for ethnic minorities. Discuss how you would provide competent nursing care to a diverse group.

7. Generate a group discussion during class about beliefs and values regarding mentally ill persons who are in a correctional institution.

Characteristics of the Client Population

- The Mentally Ill Offender

- Gender Issues

- Cultural Issues

Conflicting Convictions: Custody and Caring

- Nurse-Client Relationship

- Treatment Setting

- Professional Role Definition

  ▾ The role of the nurse in correctional settings includes but is not limited to assessing, planning, implementing, evaluating, and coordinating nursing care consistent with the needs of the inmate population.

- Societal Norms

CHAPTER 34: The Grieving Process: Dealing with Loss

Case Presentation

Ms. X. is a 59-year-old semi-retired woman with the equivalent of an eighth grade education. She was referred to the community mental health clinic for treatment after the death of her husband, who had struggled with a chronic and lengthy illness. They had been married for 30 years and raised and educated four children. She has maintained active contact with all of her children as well as with the numerous friends that she had known over the years both in the workplace and through social activities. She did not report any history of psychological difficulty prior to the death of her husband. Immediately after his death, Ms. X. became depressed, developed symptoms of insomnia, loss of appetite, low activity level, poor concentration, and a numb feeling in the head. She complained that her finances were limited because of the costly funeral and the limited resources left by her late husband. She reported that she has strong feelings of anger and bitterness, not only because of her husband's death but also because her children live far away. She felt a strong need for security and dependence. She indicated that frequent thoughts about her husband's death interfered with her daily functioning both at home and while she was working at her part-time job. She stated, "I've spent so many years caring for him, life is empty without him." During the initial interview, Ms. X. stated that she would not consider suicide because it was against her religious orientation. She cried when she talked about her past life experiences. She revealed that during her childhood and adolescence, the family frequently moved from one location to another because of her father's inability to find permanent employment. She stated that she had suffered many losses, which included friends, a favorite cat, a bedroom of her own, and the death of her father when she was 15 years old. She said that her family never talked about her father's death, and she thinks that these experiences have left a permanent scar and that they impede her ability to deal with the loss of her husband. Ms. X. agreed to see the clinical nurse specialist for treatment of depression and to gain insight into the grief process. The treatment began with a psychoeducational component and focused on earlier losses and trauma. During the sessions agreed upon, Ms. X. was able to accept the reality and pain of the loss, connect past experiences with her reaction to her husband's death, adjust to the environment without her husband, and move beyond her monetary deficits.

Critical Thinking Issues

1. Identify the significant assessment findings.

2. Using the descriptive data, develop a plan for nursing interventions.

3. Identify the stages of grief.

4. Examine the differences between normal and complicated grief.

5. What are the short- and long-term goals for a person in the grieving state?

Student Activities

1. Review the symptoms of normal grief and major depression.

2. List six differences between normal grief and depression.

Normal Grief	**Major Depression**
a._____	a._____
_____	_____
b._____	b._____
_____	_____
c._____	c._____
_____	_____
d._____	d._____
_____	_____
e._____	e._____
_____	_____
f._____	f._____
_____	_____

3. Interview a person who has experienced major losses, and determine how his or her coping strategies helped through the grieving process.

4. Divide into groups of four or five students. Each group should discuss beliefs and values regarding death and dying. The groups should share the information with the class.

5. The grieving process that is experienced by other cultures may be different. Discuss how different cultures view death and dying.

The Grieving Process: Dealing With Loss

- Characteristics of the Grieving Process

- Types of Grieving Experienced by Clients

- The Context of Nursing Care in the Grieving Process

  ▾ The Nurse–Client Relationship

  ▾ Assisting Clients in the Grieving Process

CHAPTER 35: Future Trends

Case Presentation

Jane, RN, an entrepreneur, established a virtual organization—a network of services that integrate a closer relationship between psychiatric mental health nursing care and the primary nursing care system. This innovative system provides speed of communication and a comprehensive continuum of services through an Internet system and a team of professionals. Databases are shared with the clinicians working with their clients. Direct service is provided to urban and rural populations and includes home care, day programs, schools, factories, floating and cruise ship hotels/condominiums, retirement residences, and shopping center clinics. Services provided throughout the regional marketplace include education, promotion of self-care, and working with community leaders and politicians to stimulate lifestyle changes. Policies related to reimbursement for care were changed to accommodate those persons in great need. The Internet service provides clients with a resource for information about psychiatric illnesses. Owing to a change in global lifestyle, health-care policies, socioeconomic shifts, managed care, population movement, and cultural, political and environmental limitations, Jane is challenged and is at the forefront responding to the health-care environment and initiating and implementing change.

Critical Thinking Issues

1. Discuss societal changes and how psychiatric mental health nursing will be challenged during the next millennium.

2. Discuss the implications of multiprofessionals delivering psychiatric mental health services.

3. Analyze the future roles of the psychiatric generalist and the clinical nurse specialist.

4. What are the implications for the future nursing workforce related to the psychiatric mental health nurse?

Student Activities

1. Assign each student to browse the Internet for information related to the delivery of psychiatric mental health nursing. This information may be obtained from a school of nursing's home page or from a psychiatric home health agency's home page.

2. Generate a class discussion related to establishing shared databases. Discuss the importance of such information banks.

3. Discuss multistate licensure and its effect on the delivery of psychiatric mental health nursing.

4. Discuss the importance of political involvement and the opportunities for nurses in the political arena.

5. Invite a nurse who is a member of the state or federal legislative body to speak to the class.

The Present and Future of Psychiatric Mental Health Care: Managed Care

- The Fee-for-Service Delivery System

- The Managed Care Delivery System

Effects of Managed Care on Psychiatric Mental Health Care Delivery

Opportunities for Psychiatric Nurses

- Roles for the Psychiatric Generalist Nurse

- Roles for the Psychiatric Clinical Nurse Specialist (CNS)

Challenges for Future Psychiatric Nurses